GOD'S
AMAZING
PHARMACY

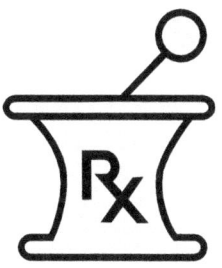

Food is a powerful chemical.   Food is as powerful as any medicine. Food can cause/ prevent/ and/or -heal - medical diseases. Food can successfully prevent, treat and therefore heal many medical diseases such as Obesity, Diabetes, Arthritis, Eye Disease, Hypertension, Heart Disease (Hypercholesterolemia - Hypertriglyceridemia), Kidney Disease, Sleep Disorders, Depression, Fibromyalgia, and Neurological Diseases, etc.

Food can <u>cause Cancer</u>. Food can <u>prevent Cancer</u>.

Hippocrates once said:
"Let your food be your Medicine and Let your Medicine be your Food".
Hippocrates got it right 2000 years ago.

God's Word (3 John 1 & 2) states:

"Beloved, I pray that in all respects you may prosper and be in good health, just as your soul prospers."

God has truly provided everything we need for good health and life!

God's Amazing Pharmacy

The knowledge you gain from reading this book will help you select a more natural way to improve your health and even heal many , if not all, of your medical diseases or illnesses. This knowledge will also inspire you to eat more nutritiously knowing that you are preventing many of the long term age-related metabolic diseases that have become pandemic in America today. You will be able to enjoy a better quality of life – longer. This healthy life style depends entirely on the types of nutrients (foods) you choose to eat on a regular, daily basis.

"MY PEOPLE PERISH FOR LACK OF KNOWLEDGE"
Hosea 4:6

KNOWLEDGE - IS - POWERFUL!

A healthy body is something to be cherished. In fact, it is more valuable than wealth.

Other Books by

Denise Marks, M.D.

Food is Your Best Medicine

The Importance of the Sugar/Fiber Ratio

GOD'S AMAZING PHARMACY

For written inquiries, use the address below

AtoZ Publishing Group, LLC

40 Plaza Way, 8-132, Mountain Home, AR 72653

http//www.atozpublishinggroup.com

Published in the United States of America

DEDICATION

I want to dedicate this book to my two sons, Jason and Justin Sharbono, who sacrificed the time I spent away studying to become a medical doctor.

Table of Contents

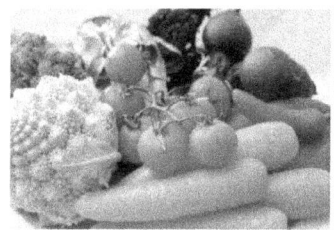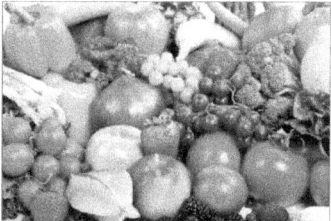

GOD'S AMAZING PHARMACY

PREFACE

I write this book, not only for the millions of Americans who may have a medical problem, but also for all who may not be aware of the medicinal value of food. Medicine is not only defined as a treatment for illness and disease, it is now understood that <u>medicine is for the prevention of illness and disease.</u>

Even laughter is a medicine because research found it to boost the immune system. Exercise is good medicine for its cardio-vascular stimulation, muscle toning and flexibility and expelling toxins and for giving you a feeling of well-being, all immune boosters. To express a positive attitude towards life is not only good medicine for you: it is also good medicine for those in contact with you.

<u>But the most important medicine, especially for the prevention of illness and disease, is our diet.</u>

It means supplying proper hydration and the needed nutrients to effectively maintain a state of well-being. <u>This medicine called nutrition</u> amplifies the significance of our eating habits and our lifestyle.

It is a well established fact that most of our modern-day medical problems are due to the foods we eat. Foods contain nutrients and nutrients are medicinal chemicals that must be supplied by the diet – daily - in order for the body to be in good health.

A healthy human body is a remarkable work of art and should be nurtured, cared for and cherished. However, many Americans are not taking good care of their body simply by

1

not feeding their body the high-quality nutrient's it needs and deserves. If the body does not receive the proper building blocks it needs for energy, maintenance, or repair, it is only a matter of time before it fails to run in an efficient, healthy manner. Good health for living life to the fullest depends on the body receiving the full range of nutrients it needs on a regular, daily basis.

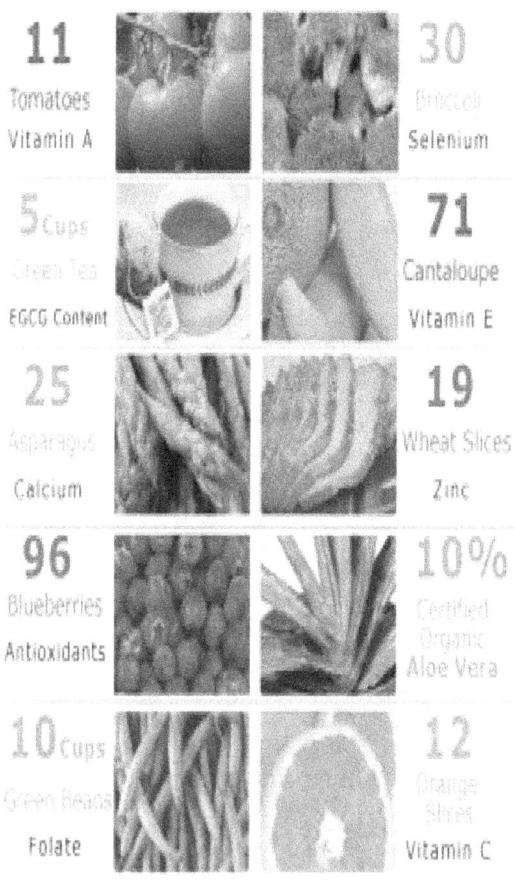

11 Tomatoes Vitamin A	**30** Broccoli Selenium
5 Cups Green Tea EGCG Content	**71** Cantaloupe Vitamin E
25 Asparagus Calcium	**19** Wheat Slices Zinc
96 Blueberries Antioxidants	**10%** Certified Organic Aloe Vera
10 Cups Green Beans Folate	**12** Orange Slices Vitamin C

The human body is actually the vessel of "your mind and soul". God, in His Word (3 John 1 & 2), states this concept another way. "Beloved, I pray that in all respects you may prosper and be in good health, just as your soul prospers." A healthy mind and body is something to be nurtured and cherished. In fact, a healthy mind and body is more valuable than wealth.

Hippocrates, a well known scientist, stated 2,000 years ago:

> **"Let food be your medicine and let medicine be your food."**

He was teaching people of that era the value of food in the care of the human body. He got it right 2000 years ago and this truth still applies to our health today.

Food is a powerful chemical. Food is as powerful as any medicine. Food can either heal or cause disease.

Food can successfully treat, correct and in many cases heal many of our metabolic medical diseases, such as:

Obesity/Overweight, Diabetes, Hypertension, Kidney Disease, Coronary Heart Disease, (Hypercholesterolemia / Hypertriglyceridemia), Depression, Arthritis, Fibromyalgia, Eye Disease, Neurological Disease, etc.

Most noteworthy, is the fact that "Food can cause Cancer and food can prevent Cancer".

Food contains many different nutrients. These nutrients are medicinal chemicals that are needed by the body for the many different, yet specific, biochemical processes that are going on daily (in fact minute by minute) and are required in order for the body to optimally function and maintain good health - free of disease.

Food can actually be used to treat or heal whatever ails your body *instead of many of the expensive pharmaceutical medicines that are basically "copy-cats" of a plant's biochemical structure that does the same thing medically speaking, but the side effect profile of these man-made medicines is usually worse and in fact cause more medical problems than if the disease was left untreated.*

This knowledge of the pharmaceutical relationship of food, especially plant nutrients, to the healing process of medical diseases is applied to the treatment of many of the age-related metabolic diseases.

For example, just by knowing which foods contain the right nutrients, (i.e., medicinal chemicals), you can repair or heal damaged insulin receptors.

These damaged insulin receptors cause "Insulin Resistance" and are known to be the root cause of type 2 diabetes as well as many other metabolic medical diseases such as: i.e. arthritis, hypertension, heart disease, and some cancers, etc.

Also, by understanding the root cause (inflammation) of these metabolic diseases you can choose to eat the foods that contain the specific (healing) nutrients that will maintain those biochemical processes and prevent these diseases from even beginning.

Many biochemical processes are affected by the type of food as well as the pharmaceutical drugs you consume, especially those biochemical processes that take place in the liver.

An example of one of these biochemical processes is gluconeogenesis. **Gluconeogenesis** is called "the fat burning process" 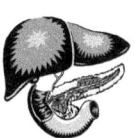 because the liver uses this process to convert triglyceride molecules (body fat) into glucose (sugar) molecules for energy.

The drug, Metformin / Glucophage that is prescribed the most by physicians for newly diagnosed type 2 diabetes: blocks gluconeogensis.

Also, high glycemic, sweet tasting foods and non-nutritive artificial sweeteners are known to block or muck-up this "fat burning process".

 The next thing that happens is that triglyceride and cholesterol levels become elevated causing more medical problems. A malfunction or blocking of this biochemical process, gluconeogensis, leads to a whole host the age-related medical diseases: i.e., weight gain, obesity, eye disease, heart disease, hypercholesterolemia, hypertriglyceridemia, kidney disease, arthritis, and some cancers, etc.

Research has revealed that more than two thirds of all deaths in the United States are diet related. More than 50% of all deaths are caused from coronary occlusion, blockage of the blood flow to the heart and/or the brain. These are all preventable deaths.

Basically all coronary occlusion can be eliminated by 97% through a vegetarian diet. A huge number of American's are dying of cancer every day. And yet there is overwhelming evidence that a nutritious diet, free of processed foods, is the best prevention for this horrible modern day metabolic disease.

My hope is that the information in this book will inspire you to make healthier "food" choices that will result in a healthier and happier you.

DENISE MARKS, M.D.

INTRODUCTION: FOOD CONTAINS NUTRIENTS AND NUTRIENTS ARE MEDICINES!

Food contains nutrients and these nutrients can and do act as medicinal chemicals. These nutrients can be used by the body to not only make hormones, maintain good health and provide energy, but also they can be used to prevent and heal the body of specific medical diseases! All nutrients can be divided into macronutrients and/or micronutrients.

Nutrients, Daily value, Function, Sources

NUTRIENT	DAILY VALUE*	FUNCTION	
Protein	16g	Important for growth and development of your child; also important for making and repairing cells	Good sources include poultry, meat, fish, beans, nuts, dairy products and soy
Fiber	NA	Important for preventing constipation; also helps decrease the risk of Type 2 Diabetes, heart disease and high cholesterol later in life	Good sources include fresh fruits with the skin on, dried fruit, vegetables, beans/legumes, whole grains such as brown rice and whole wheat bread
Calcium	800 mg	Important for strong bones and teeth; helps with muscle functioning, blood clotting, nerve transmission	Good sources include dairy products, leafy green vegetables, calcium fortified foods such as orange juice and tofu
Iron	10 mg	Important for your child's growth; also important for forming hemoglobin to carry oxygen through the body, a lack of it can lead to fatigue	Good sources include poultry, meat, fish, eggs, raisins, leafy green vegetables, beans and enriched grains
Vitamin A	2500 IU	Important for eyesight, growth, functioning of the immune system and healthy skin	Good sources include dark green vegetables such as spinach, orange fruits and vegetables such as sweet potatoes and papayas, dairy products fortified with vitamin A such as milk, eggs
Vitamin C	40 mg	Important for decreasing risk of colds, infections, recurrent ear infections; wound healing; keeping gums, skin and muscles healthy; aids in brain function; also an antioxidant	Good sources include citrus fruits, broccoli, strawberries, tomatoes, bell pepers, kale
Vitamin D	400 IU	Important for strong bones and teeth because it helps absorb calcium; also important in immune function	Good sources include milk fortified with vitamin D, fatty fish, egg yolks and the sun (depending on latitude and time of year)

Daily Values are Based on Children Under 4 years of age

Macronutrients are the caloric nutrients. Macronutrients are carbohydrates, proteins, or fats

Carbohydrates are either simple or complex carbohydrates.

Proteins are made up of amino acid molecules.

Essential amino acids are those types of amino acids the body cannot make on its own and nonessential amino acids are those types of amino acids the body can make even if the foods consumed do not contain protein.

Fats are either unsaturated or saturated fats, mono-, di-, or tri-glycerides, and/or omega 3 or omega 6 fatty acids. Trans-fats also fit the definition of a saturated fat. [Trans-fats are man-made fats by forcing Hydrogen gas (hydrogenation) into natural oils]. Some examples of foods that contain these hydrogenated oils are margarine and shortening and products made with these fats. Interesting is the fact that hydrogenated oils are just a few steps away from being a plastic molecule.

For example, if you were to burn at very high temperatures a stick of margarine it would turn into a glob of plastic. Hydrogenated oils are trans-fats and are more likely to cause medical problems than butter or lard, i.e., natural saturated fats.

Even cholesterol, a waxy-like substrate, is considered a fat at times. Cholesterol can be a good fat if it is bonded to the good lipoprotein (HDL). The difference in its character depends on which lipoprotein hooks up to cholesterol in the first place and carries it through the blood stream. That difference usually depends on the amount of glucose (sugar) and insulin that are also in the blood stream.

Micronutrients are non-caloric nutrients. Micronutrients are: vitamins, minerals, and/or phytonutrients.

Vitamins are those organic micronutrients that the body cannot make and therefore must be supplied daily from the foods we eat.

Minerals are elements that the body needs in order to complete or make happen the many biochemical processes needed by the body to make structures (i.e. cells, cell membranes, bones, blood, hormones, neurotransmitters, etc.).

Phytonutrients are basically the organic nutrient components of plants: especially, fruits, vegetables, nuts, seeds, legumes, herbs, spices and teas.

Phytonutrients are thought to have medicinal properties that promote good health.

Scientifically, they are classified as carotenoids, polyphenols (flavonoids and non-flavonoids, lignans), indoles, inositols, etc. All 'food' nutrients are important, but the micronutrients, (especially the phytonutrients), are actually the most important nutrients needed by the body for the maintenance of good health and/or the prevention of most diseases.

Phytonutrients either contain anti-oxidants that neutralize free radicals or they contain anti-inflammatory agents that heal swollen or damaged cells structures.

Vitamins: The following is a list of micronutrients that are recognized as vitamins.

- Vitamin A (Retinol or Carotenoids), Sweet Potatoes, Spinach, Carrots, Eggs, Fish and Liver
- Vitamin B1(thiamine), B2(riboflavin), B3(niacin), B5(pantothenic acid), B6(pyridoxine), B7(biotin), B9(folic acid),B12(cyanocobalamine), found in most meats and vegetables.
- Vitamin C (ascorbic acid), Citrus and Non-Citrus Fruit, and Vegetables, i.e., peppers& kale
- Vitamin D (Ergocalciferol or Cholecalciferal), Milk and Milk products, Salmon and Oranges
- Vitamin E (Tocopherol or Tocotrienol), Nuts and Wheat Germ
- Vitamin K (Phylloquinone or Menaquinone), Green leafy veg. - Kale, Beet & Mustard greens
- Vitamin Q (Coenzyme Q10 or CoQ10). A necessary vitamin for strong healthy muscles. a type of vitamin needed to be supplemented by individuals placed on statin drugs, (cholesterol lowering drugs). This is because the body's biochemical machinery for making natural Coenzyme Q-10 is blocked by all "statin" drugs.

Minerals: Some of the most common elements (minerals) needed by the body are:

1) calcium - gives structure and strength to bones, teeth, muscles, and enzymes and nerves.
2) chromium - necessary for proper function of insulin, cellular metabolism.
3) copper - plays an important role in nerve function, bone growth, fetal development, formation of blood cells, heart and muscle movement and tone and development of the brain and nervous system.
4) iodine - necessary for the production of the thyroid hormone
5) iron - carries oxygen through the body, helps regulate temperature and cognitive function
6) magnesium - functions in muscle contraction, prevents preterm labor, nervous disorders & stress
7) sodium - an electrolyte that helps maintain the balance of fluid, transmission of nerve impulses, regulates temperature, blood pressure and prevents seizures.
8) manganese - acts as an anti-oxidant, co-factor with enzymes & heal tissue wounds
9) phosphorus - plays a role in production of enzymes, hormones, pH balance, and energy
10)potassium - acts as an electrolyte and functions in nerve conduction & muscle contraction
11) selenium - helps protect cells from free radicals, necessary for thyroid and immune function
12) zinc - immune response, brain function, binds to DNA, metabolism and ability to reproduce, growth gestation, disease prevention, and helps control release of hormones and transmission of nerve impulses

Phytonutrients: There are basically seven common groups of phytonutrients. These groups are 1. Phenolic nutrients, 2. Terpenes (isoprenoids) include carotenoids and monterpenoids, , 3. Betalains, 4. Organosulfides (the onion and garlic family), 5. Indoles, (other sulfur containing nutrients, i.e. glucosinolates found in the cabbage family), 6. Protein inhibitors and 7 other organic acids. Some of the common classes of phytonutrients include:

*1. Phenolic (Phenols) Phytonutrients
  Natural monophenols
    Apiole – parsley, celery leaf.
    Carnosol – rosemary, sage
    Carvacrol – oregano, thyme, pepperwort, wild bergamot.
    Dillapiole – dill, fennel root.
    Rosemarinol – rosemary.
  Flavonoids (polyphenols) – red, blue, purple pigments.
    Flavonols
      Quercetin – red and yellow onions, tea, wine, apples, cranberries, buckwheat, beans.
      Gingerol – ginger.
      Kaempferol – tea, strawberries, gooseberries, cranberries, grapefruit, apples, peas.
      Brassicates broccoli, kale, Brussels sprouts, cabbage.
      Myricetin – grapes, red wine, berries, walnuts.
      Rutin – citrus fruits, oranges, lemons, limes, grapefruit, berries, peaches, apples, asparagus, buckwheat, parsley, tomatoes, apricots, rhubarb, tea.
      Isorhamnetin – red turnip, goldenrod, mustard leaf, ginkgo biloba.
    Flavanones
      Hesperidin – citrus fruits.
      Naringenin – citrus fruits.
      Silybin – blessed milk thistle.
    Flavones
      Acacetin – Robinia pseudoacacia, Turnera diffusa.
      Apigenin – chamomile, celery, parsley.

Chrysin – Passiflora caerulea, Pleurotus ostreatus, Oroxylum indicum.

Diosmetin – Vicia.

Tangeritin – tangerine and other citrus peels.

Luteolin – beets, artichokes, celery, carrots, celeriac, rutabaga, parsley, mint, chamomile, lemongrass, chrysanthemum

Flavan-3-ols

Catechins – white tea, green tea, black tea, grapes, wine, apple juice, cocoa, lentils, black-eyed peas.

Epigallocatechin gallate (EGCG) – green tea:

Theaflavin – black tea:

Theaflavin-3-gallate – black tea:

Thearubigins

Flavonals (Anthocyanins) red wine, many red, purple or blue fruits and vegetables.

Pelargonidin – bilberry, raspberry, strawberry.

Peonidin – bilberry, blueberry, cherry, cranberry, peach.

Cyanidin – red apple & pear, bilberry, blackberry, blueberry, cherry, cranberry, peach, plum, hawthorn, loganberry, cocoa.

Delphinidin – bilberry, blueberry, eggplant.

Malvidin – bilberry, blueberry.

Isoflavones (phytoestrogens) (nonflavonoid)

Daidzein (formononetin) – soy, chickpeas, peanuts, other legumes.

Genistein (biochanin A) – soy, alfalfa sprouts, red clover, chickpeas, peanuts, other legumes.

Glycitein – soy.

Coumestans (phytoestrogens)

Coumestrol –soy, peas, Brussels sprouts.

Prenylflavonoids

6-prenylnaringenin - grapefruit

Xanthohumol

Phenolic acids

Ellagic acid – walnuts, strawberries, cranberries, blackberries, guava, grapes.

Gallic acid – tea, mango, strawberries, rhubarb, soy.

Salicylic acid – peppermint, licorice.

Tannic acid – nettles, tea, berries.

Vanillin – vanilla beans, cloves.

Capsaicin – chili peppers.

Curcumin – turmeric, mustard.

Hydroxycinnamic acids

Caffeic acid –, artichoke, pear, basil, thyme, oregano, apple, olive oil.

Chlorogenic acid – echinacea, strawberries, pineapple, coffee, sunflower, blueberries.

Cinnamic acid – cinnamon, aloe.

Ferulic acid – oats, rice, artichoke, orange, pineapple, apple, peanut.

Coumarin – citrus fruits, maize.

Lignans (phytoestrogens) – seeds (flax, sesame, pumpkin, sunflower, poppy), whole grains (rye, oats, barley), bran (wheat, oat, rye), fruits (particularly berries) and vegetables.

Silymarin – artichokes, milk thistle.

Matairesinol – flax seed, sesame seed, rye bran, oat bran, poppy seed, strawberries,
blackcurrants, broccoli.

Secoisolariciresinol – flax seeds, sunflower seeds, sesame seeds, pumpkin, strawberries,
blueberries, cranberries, zucchini, blackcurrant, carrots.

Pinoresinol and lariciresinol – sesame seed, Brassica vegetables

Tyrosol esters

Tyrosol – olive oil

Hydroxytyrosol – olive oil

Oleocanthal – olive oil

Oleuropein – olive oil

Stilbenoids

Resveratrol – grape skins and seeds, wine, nuts, peanuts.

Pterostilbene – grapes, blueberries

Piceatannol – grapes

Punicalagins – pomegranates

Alkylresorcinols – wholegrain wheat, rye and barley

*2.Terpenes (isoprenoids)

Carotenoids (tetraterpenoids)

Carotenes - orange pigments

α-Carotene –carrots, pumpkins, maize, tangerine, orange.

β-Carotene –dark, leafy greens and red, orange and yellow fruits and vegetables.

Lycopene tomatoes, grapefruit, watermelon, guava, apricots, carrots, autumn olive.

Phytofluene – star fruit, sweet potato, orange.

Phytoene – sweet potato, orange.

Xanthophylls - yellow pigments.

Canthaxanthin – paprika.

Cryptoxanthin to vitamin A, mango, orange, papaya, peaches, avocado, pea, grapefruit, kiwi.

Zeaxanthin –spinach, kale, turnip greens, maize, eggs, red pepper, pumpkin, oranges.

Astaxanthin – microalge, yeast, krill, shrimp, salmon, lobsters, and some crabs

Lutein – spinach, greens, lettuce, eggs, red pepper, pumpkin, mango, papaya, oranges, kiwi, peaches, squash, prunes, sweet potatoes, honeydew melon, rhubarb, plum, avocado, pear.

Monoterpenes

Limonene – oils of citrus, cherries, spearmint, dill, garlic, celery, maize, rosemary, ginger, basil.

Perillyl alcohol – citrus oils, caraway, mints.

Saponins – soybeans, beans, other legumes, maize, alfalfa.

Lipids

Phytosterols almonds, cashews, peanuts, sesame and sunflower seeds, maize, soybeans, vegetable oils.

Campesterol - buckwheat.

Beta Sitosterol avocados, rice and wheat germ, corn oils, peanuts, soybeans, basil, buckwheat.

Stigmasterol – buckwheat.

Tocopherols (vitamin E)

Omega-3, 6, 9 fatty acids –(ALA and LA) dark-green leafy vegetables, grains, legumes, nuts.

Gamma-linolenic acid – evening primrose, borage, blackcurrant.
Triterpenoid
Oleanolic acid - pokeweed, honey mesquite, garlic, java, apple, cloves, other Syzygium species.
Ursolic acid - apples, basil, bilberries, cranberries, peppermint, lavender, oregano, thyme, prunes.
Betulinic acid - Ber tree, white birch, tropical carnivorous plants Triphyophyllum peltatum
Moronic acid - Rhus javanica (a sumac), mistletoe

*3. Betalains
Betalains (Betaxanthins) beets, Sicilian prickly pear.
*4. Organosulfides
Dithiolthiones (isothiocyanates) Sulphoraphane – Brassicates.
Polysulfides (allium compounds) Allyl methyl trisulfide – garlic, onions, leeks, chives, shallots.
Sulfides Diallyl disulfide – garlic, onions, leeks, chives, shallots.

*5. Indoles, glucosinolates/ sulfur compounds
Indole-3-carbinol – cabbage, kale, brussels sprouts, rutabaga, mustard greens, broccoli.
Sulforaphane - broccoli, cauliflower, brussels sprouts, cabbages
3,3'-Diindolylmethane or DIM - broccoli family, brussels sprouts, cabbage, kale
Sinigrin - broccoli family, brussels sprouts, black mustard
Allicin - garlic
Alliin - garlic
Allyl isothiocyanate - horseradish, mustard, wasabi
Piperine - black pepper
Syn-propanethial-S-oxide - cut onions.

*6. Protein inhibitors

Protease inhibitors – soy, seeds, legumes, potatoes, eggs, cereals.

*7. Other organic acids

Oxalic acid – orange, spinach, rhubarb, tea and coffee, banana, ginger, almond, sweet potato,

bell pepper.

Phytic acid (inositol hexaphosphate) cereals, nuts, sesame seeds, soybeans, wheat, pumpkin,

beans, almonds.

Tartaric acid – apricots, apples, sunflower, avocado, grapes, tamarind.

Anacardic acid - cashews, mangoes.

CHAPTER 1 GOD'S PHARMACY IS AMAZING!!

The definition of a medicine is: any agent or substance used in the treatment or prevention of disease or illness or in the relief or prevention of pain. The definition of pharmacy is: the art or practice of preparing medical drugs or agents used in the treatment of disease or in the relief of pain.

Foods contain nutrients and nutrients are the chemicals that actually treat, prevent or heal diseases, illnesses or relieve pain. Therefore, by definition of a medicine, food nutrients are medicines. Hippocrates, a well known scientist 2000 years ago, got it right when he said "Let food be your medicine and let medicine by your food".

Foods contain nutrients that can be used by the body to prevent diseases, heal diseases, cure infections and help prevent or relieve pain. Therefore, nutrients are natural medicines by the strictest sense of the definition.

The best representation of a natural agent that can relieve pain and therefore is a natural medicine is the opium plant. It still relieves pain in its natural state with no side effects & no end-organ damage.

Pharmaceutical pain relievers usually contain Tylenol and/or Ibuprofen as well as other additives so it can be made into a 'pill' to be patented. All man-made drugs have side-effects either because of the fixed concentrated dose or the additives used to make the drug.

These drugs are known to cause other problems and even other diseases. Natural food nutrients don't have additives, unless they are processed foods, therefore they have fewer negative side effects than man-made drugs.

GOD'S PHARMACY!

From the beginning of time God has supplied us with good things that will not only heal our diseases but also keep us healthy and well. Food nutrients (medicinal chemicals found in food) are what I call "God's pharmacy". From the beginning of time, God has made these powerful chemicals available to sustain us as well as heal our bodies. God also provided great clues as to which food would help or heal certain organs or cells in our body. The following is a list of some foods that have nutrients that contribute to the health of specific organs or tissues in the body.

1.   CARROTS, a sliced carrot looks like the human eye. The radiating lines in the cut section of the carrot look just like the pupil and iris of the human eye. And yes, science does show carrots greatly enhance the function of the eye.

2.   AVOCADOES, PEARS, AND EGGPLANTS: these foods target the health and function of the womb and cervix of the female body – and yes, they look just like the womb. If women would eat just one of these foods three times a week, their hormones would be or become balanced, and they would be able to shed unwanted pounds, prevent cervical cancers &

increase the production of sex hormones. HOW PROFOUND IS THIS NEXT TRIVIA? **"It takes exactly nine (9) months to grow an avocado from blossom to ripened fruit"**.

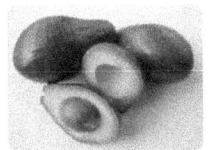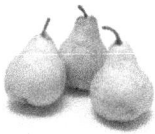

3.   CELERY, BOK CHOY, OR RHUBARB: and many more stalk- like foods look and structurally act like bones. These foods specifically target bone strength. Bones are 23% sodium and these foods are 23% sodium. If you don't get enough sodium in your diet, the body pulls it from the bones, thus making them weak. These foods also replenish the skeletal needs of the body.

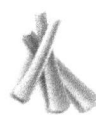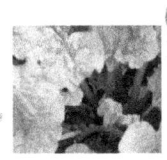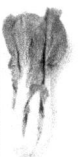

4.   FIGS: figs are full of seeds and hang in twos when they grow on the fig tree. Figs increase the mobility of male sperm and increase the numbers of sperm and will overcome male sterility. And as you can see they look like testicles.

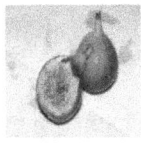

5.

GRAPES: grapes hang in a cluster that has the shape of the heart. Each grape looks like a blood cell and research today shows that grapes are also a profound heart and blood vitalizing food.

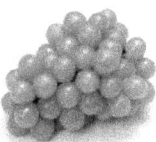

6. KIDNEY BEANS: these odd-shaped powerful beans are full of nutrients. They actually heal and help maintain kidney function and yes, they look exactly like the human kidneys.

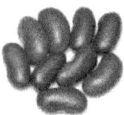

7. OLIVES: olives look like ovaries and they actually promote the health and function of the ovaries. They are even the same size as a normal adult ovary.

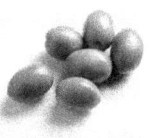

8. ONIONS, AND GARLIC: onions and garlic look similar to the body's cells. Today's research shows onions help clear waste materials from all of the body cells.

They even produce tears which wash the epithelial layers of the eyes. A working companion, Garlic, also helps eliminate waste materials as well as the dangerous "free radicals" that cause most of our age-related medical disease.

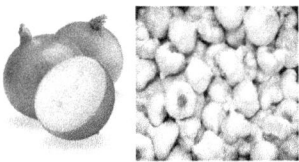

9.   ORANGES, GRAPEFRUITS, AND OTHER CITRUS FRUITS, look just like the mammary glands of the female and actually assist the health of the breasts and the movement of lymph in and out of the breast tissues.

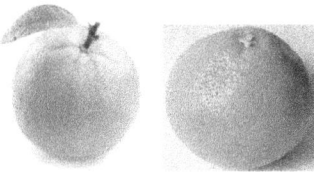

10.   SWEET POTATOES, look like the pancreas. Sweet potatoes actually balance the "glucose to insulin ratio" and prevent type 2 diabetes.

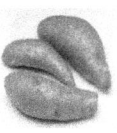

11.   TOMATOES: a tomato has four chambers and is red. The heart has four chambers and is red. Research shows tomatoes are loaded with lycopine, which is a very good heart and blood nutrient.

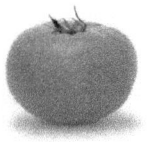 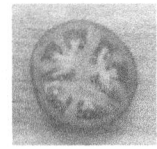

12. <u>WALNUTS</u>: a walnut looks like a little brain, a left and right hemisphere, upper cerebrums and lower cerebellums. Even the wrinkles or folds on the nut are just like the neo-cortex. We now know walnuts help develop more than three dozen neuro-transmitters necessary for brain function.

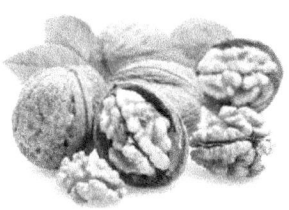

CHAPTER 2   NUTRIENTS ARE MEDICINES

Fruit in general, is an excellent source of many vital anti-oxidant and anti-inflammatory nutrients. Note: anti-oxidant nutrients neutralize free radicals before they cause damage and disease and anti-inflammatory nutrients reduce swelling and fix the damage caused by free radicals, toxins and infective agents that cause disease.

Anti-oxidant and anti-inflammatory nutrients are the vitamins such as vitamin A, some of the B vitamins, and vitamin C, and phyto-nutrients such as carotenoids, flavonoids, poly-phenols, phenols, lignans, inositol and indoles to mention a few. Regular consumption of fruits as well as vegetables has been shown to offer significant protection against many chronic degenerative diseases such as: cancer, heart disease, strokes, cataracts, arthritis and even diabetes and neurological diseases.

Although fructose and other sugars are as much as one and a half times sweeter than sucrose (white sugar), they are handled by the body in a different manner. For example, in order for fructose to be utilized by the body for energy, it must first be converted into glucose during a biochemical process, **glucogenolosis**, in the liver.

 This process involves the Krebs cycle: which requires an enzyme that is found only in the liver, namely, Glyceraldehyde 3-Phosphate. Therefore, fructose initially bypasses the pancreas and thus blocks the pancreas from releasing a surge (large dose) of insulin.

As a result, blood sugar (glucose) levels do not rise as rapidly after fructose (fruit) consumption and therefore less insulin is required to process fructose compared to other simple sugars. Consuming sucrose, which is composed of one molecule of glucose and one molecule of fructose, results in an immediate elevation in blood sugar and the release of a large dose (surge) of insulin. Hyper-insulinemia, (as a result of consuming large amounts of sugar and other high glycemic foods and/or taking high doses of insulin medications), is the root cause of most of our age-related metabolic diseases.

The fact that high glucose and high doses or surges of insulin is the root cause of most of our age-related metabolic diseases is a very important reason to consume less high glycemic foods.

While most diabetics cannot tolerate sucrose, most diabetics can tolerate moderate amounts of fruit and fructose without loss of blood sugar control. In fact, fruit is much better tolerated and has a lower glycemic index than white bread (the standard) and other refined carbohydrates.

Since fruit contains a fair amount of the natural fruit sugar, mainly fructose and a smaller percentage of glucose depending on the fruit, it is generally recommended by nutritionist to limit our intake of fruit to four servings of fruits or two 8 oz glasses of fresh (unprocessed) fruit juice a day, again depending on the fruit. For instance, apples have less fruit sugar than grapes or peaches pound for pound.

If you suffer from hypoglycemia, diabetes, candidacies or gout, it is probably best for you to eat fruit in its whole form or drink fresh fruit juice with food or dilute it with an equal amount of pure water. Eating whole fruit provides more fiber and drinking diluted juice decreases the rate at which sugar enters your blood stream compared to drinking concentrated fruit drinks. This is especially true if the juice drinks are processed meaning they contain a significant amount of high fructose corn syrup. The fiber in whole fruit and diluted natural juices prevents a surge of insulin from being released from the pancreas.

Since fruit contains fructose in its natural form, consuming a serving of fruit or fruit juice at least 30 minutes before dinner may result in significantly fewer calories being consumed during the meal. Eating fruit as an appetizer before your meal would be one way to prevent a surge of insulin or hyperinsulinemia, (i.e., large amount of insulin in the blood stream).

When fewer calories (especially fewer high glycemic carbohydrates) are consumed during the meal, **weight loss is much easier to achieve**. Also, fruit makes an excellent between-meal snack because it is packed full of anti-oxidant and anti-inflammatory nutrients which not only prevent but also heal many medical diseases.

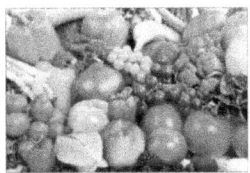

Fruits contain anti-oxidants that act like medicinal agents that can heal disease!

<u>Vegetables</u> provide the broadest range of nutrients of any class of food. Vegetables provide: natural water, fiber, minerals, vitamins and phyto-nutrients, such as carotenes, flavonoids and indoles just to mention a few.

Vegetables are rich sources of vitamins, minerals, phytonutrients, carbohydrates and protein: and the very little fat they contain is in the form of healthy fats, the essential fatty acids. The presence of many nutrients in <u>vegetables provides good health and healing to the body</u>. Vegetables provide many of the essential amino acids that the body needs grow, repair and build protein and to survive. A simple meal of spinach, beans, and whole grain rice is a great way to treat your body right. Vegetables give us a natural feeling of liveliness and energy to be more active as well as help in the healing and/or repair of damaged, infected or inflamed tissues, cells and cell receptors each day.

Vegetables help in protecting our body against cancers, diabetes and heart diseases, etc. Vegetables also add wonderful flavors to our food. Almost all vegetables are low in fat and calories.

Vegetables do not contain cholesterol.

Also, many of them are great sources of fiber that prevent the absorption of both dietary cholesterol and sugars. The high levels of fiber in vegetables keep the digestive system healthier: allowing you to avoid issues with constipation and IBS, etc. Vegetables are low in calories. This fact enables us to eat lots of vegetables with lots of nutrients without consuming excess calories.

The availability of vegetables differs from season to season. Different types of vegetables have been categorized according to their type and taste and how they develop. Some examples of the different types of vegetables that are based on growth and development patterns are:

Bulb Vegetables: Chives, Garlic, Leeks, Onions, Scallions, Shallots, Water chestnuts.
Fruit Vegetables: Avocados, Cucumbers, Eggplant, Okra, Olives, Peppers, Squash, Tomatoes, Tomatillos.
Inflorescent Vegetables: Artichokes, Broccoli, Cauliflower.
Leaf Vegetables: Arugula, Brussels sprouts, Cabbage, Chicory, Chinese cabbage, Collards, Cress, Dandelion nettles, Endive, Lamb's lettuce, Lettuce, Spinach.
Root Vegetables: Beets, Carrots, Parsnips, Radishes, Rutabaga, Turnips.

Stalk Vegetable: Asparagus, Bamboo, Celery, Chard, Fennel.
Tuber Vegetable: Jerusalem artichoke, Potato, Sweet
potato, Taro, Yam.
Legumes belong to a large family of plants having fruits that
are pods that when the pod is dry or ripe will split open and
release its seeds. These include the bean family and the
clover family. Beans are the edible seed borne in pods by
some leguminous plants. More specifically it is the pod of
that plant that can and is used as food for humans and/or
cattle, etc.
Lentils are a specific legume grown for its flat edible seeds
and for fodder. Legumes (beans) and lentils contain both
macronutrients (i.e., fats, proteins and carbohydrates)and
micronutrients (i.e., vitamins, minerals, and phyto-nutrients
such as carotenes, flavonoids, poly-phenols and indoles.

All vegetables are considered to contain low glycemic food
nutrients. Low glycemic means these nutrients do not contain
a lot of the simple carbohydrates but rather contain more of
the complex carbohydrates. Low glycemic foods will not cause
the pancreas to release a surge of insulin. Remember, a surge
of insulin causes hyperinsulinemia: which then causes insulin
resistance, the insulin dominance syndrome and diabetes,
obesity, high blood pressure, heart disease, etc.

**What is hyperinsulinemia, insulin resistance and the insulin
dominance syndrome?** Beta cells in the pancreas produce
insulin. Insulin stimulates the uptake of glucose (sugar) from
the blood into the cells of the body.

When the body's cells are resistant to the action of the insulin,
it is called insulin resistance (IR). As a result of the insulin
resistance, it takes a lot more insulin the get the glucose into
the cells and therefore the pancreas produces much more
insulin than normal.

This condition of insulin resistance can then lead to a flood of
insulin in the blood stream, hyperinsulinemia, and "the insulin

dominance syndrome." As an example, in a normal person, 1 unit of insulin might be needed to help 10 mg of glucose go into cells, but in a person whose insulin receptors are damaged, a hyperinsulinemic person, 10 units of insulin might be needed to get the same 10 mg of glucose into those cells.

 Hyperinsulinemia causes the body to operate under insulin dominance. This condition is associated with a myriad of problems including the following: (1) high triglycerides (increased risk of heart and stroke), (2) high plasminogen activator inhibitor activity, causing increased risk of blood clotting, (3) higher levels of LDL-cholesterol (the bad cholesterol) and lower levels of HDL cholesterol, (the good cholesterol lipoprotein), this ratio of high levels of LDL-cholesterol and low levels of HDL-cholesterol increases the risk of heart attack and stroke), (4) high uric acid (gout), (5) polycystic ovary syndrome, PCOS, (an endocrine disorder associated with amenorrhea, infertility, hirsutism), (6) type 2 diabetes, (7) hypertension and (8) obesity, (due to high Insulin and Leptin levels).Treating hyperinsulinemia, insulin resistance, and/or insulin dominance by eating more vegetables at every meal and in-between meal snacks can significantly reduce the health risks summarized above.

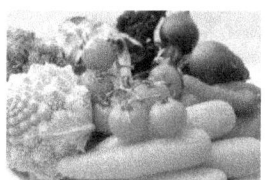

Vegetables are low glycemic nutrients that prevent hyperinsulinemia.

CHAPTER 3 FRUITS AND THEIR HEALTH BENEFITS.

1. **Apple** (Malus pumila) is a member of the rose family, along with the pear.
    Nutritional and health *info:* Apples are an excellent source of potassium, vitamin C, pectin, and other fibers. Raw apples are higher in many nutrients and phytonutrients then cooked. However, most of the apple's nutrients are in its skin. If apples are raw and unpeeled, they are excellent source of many important phytonutrients, such as ellagic acid and flavonoids (especially quercetin a well known anti-cancer phytonutrients).

    The old saying **"An apple a day keeps the doctor away"** appears to be true. An apple a day has been shown to reduce the risk of heart disease, cancer, asthma and type 2 diabetes compared to many other fruits and vegetables. Studies have shown that those who ate the most apples and other flavonoid-rich foods, such as onions and tea, were found to have a 20 percent lower risk of heart disease, diabetes and asthma than those who ate smaller amount of these foods. Researchers feel that much of apple's protective effects against heart disease and asthma are related to its high content of quercetin and other flavonoids.

    Apples are also high in pectin, a soluble fiber that has been shown to exert a number of beneficial effects. Because it is a gel forming fiber, pectin can lower cholesterol levels as well as improve the intestinal muscle's ability to better push waste through the gastrointestinal tract. In fact, adding just one large apple to the daily diet has been shown to decrease serum cholesterol by 8 to 10 percent and eating 2 large apples a day has lowered cholesterol levels by to 16 percent. It is easy to see that one or two apples a day are equal to or better then cholesterol lower drugs (statins) in lowering cholesterol. And apples are definitely less expensive and don't have the negative side-effects of these pharmaceutical drugs.

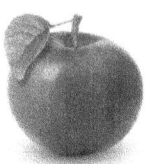

2. **Apricot** (Prunus armenaica) is classified as a 'drupe', a fleshy, one-seeded fruit containing a seed enclosed in a stony pit. It is in the same family as the almond, cherry, peach and plum.

   Nutritional and health info: Apricots are a good source of potassium, iron, and fiber as well as a good source of the following phytonutrients: carotenes, lutein, lycopine and alpha and beta-carotenes.

   Carotenes give red, orange, and yellow colors to fruits and vegetables. Apricots are particularly beneficial for preventing macular degeneration, heart disease, eye diseases, hypertension, diabetes and cancer.

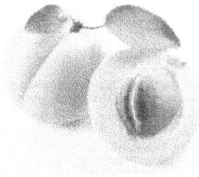

3. **Avocado** (Persea Americana). *Nutritional and health info:* Avocados are an excellent source of mono-unsaturated fatty acids, as well as potassium, vitamin E and all the B vitamins, and fiber. Avocados are high in mono-unsaturates. Their unsaturated oil content is second only to olives among fruits. The oils provided by an avocado include <u>oleic acid</u> and <u>linoleic</u>

acid. These oils are known to help lower cholesterol levels and therefore prevent as well as treat heart related diseases, i.e. hypertension, heart attack and stroke.

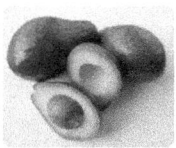

4. **Banana** (Musa sapienta). *Nutritional and health info:* Bananas are an excellent source of potassium, magnesium, fiber, and vitamin B2, B6 and B7. Bananas are packed with nutrients, especially potassium. Potassium is one of the most important electrolytes in the body, helping to regulate heart function as well as fluid balance – a key factor in regulating and lowering blood pressure and protecting against heart disease and strokes. Bananas are very soothing to the gastrointestinal tract due to their high content of pectin, a soluble fiber that not only lowers cholesterol but normalizes bowel function. Bananas are also known to heal peptic ulcers. Also, eating a banana one hour before going to bed will promote sleep and increase sleep time.

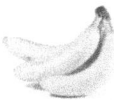

5. **Blueberry** (Vaccinium myrtillus) is a member of the Ericaceae family, along with many other berries, including huckleberries and bilberries. *Nutritional and health info:* Blueberries are an excellent source of anti-oxidant and anti-inflammatory nutrients and flavonoids, especially anthocyanidins. These antioxidant compounds are responsible for the blue, purple and red pigments in fruits. Blueberries are also a very good source of vitamin C, vitamin E and vitamin B2 (riboflavin), soluble fiber and insoluble fiber. In addition, they are a good source of

manganese. The health benefits of blueberries are due mainly to anthocyanidins. These phytonutrients exert exceptional antioxidant activity. Blueberries help protect the brain from oxidative stress and free radicals and therefore can protect against many age-related conditions, such as: Heart disease, Eye diseases and even some <u>Cancers</u> and <u>Alzheimer's</u> <u>disease</u>.

Currently, the most popular medical use of blueberries is in improving <u>vision</u> and protecting against age-related macular degeneration, the development of cataracts and glaucoma and improve night time visual acuity. Blueberries are also quite therapeutic in the treatment of varicose veins, hemorrhoids, peptic ulcers, diarrhea, constipation and promote urinary tract health. Blueberries also contain tannins, which act as astringents in the digestive system to firm up a loose stool.

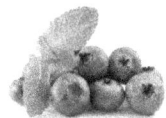

6. **Blackberries and raspberries** (Rubus idaeus) are known as "aggregate fruits" since it is made up of seed-containing fruits, called 'druplets', arranged around a hollow central cavity. *Nutritional and health info*: Raspberries are an excellent source of fiber, manganese, vitamin C, flavonoids, and ellagic acid. They are an excellent source of vitamin B2 as well as a good source of other B vitamins such as folic acid (B9), niacin (B3), pantothenic acid (B5), and pyridoxine (6). A 3 oz serving contains 52 calories, and 6 grams of fiber to 4 grams of natural sugars.

Raspberries are an excellent low-calorie, nutrient dense food. They are an excellent food for individuals with a 'sweet tooth' who are attempting to improve their quality of nutrition without increasing the caloric content of their diet. Flavonoids, mainly anthocyanidins, are responsible for the colors of raspberries as well as most of their anti-oxidant and anti-inflammatory health benefits. Note: flavonoids, and other phytonutrients act as powerful anti-oxidants. Raspberries are also an excellent source of the cancer-fighting phytonutrients, <u>ellagic acid</u>.

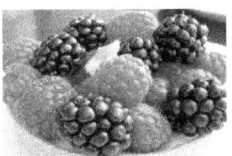

7. <u>Cantaloupe</u> (Cucumis melo reticulates) Muskmelon. Along with cucumbers, squash, gourds, and pumpkins, the cantaloupe (muskmelon) belongs to the cucurbitaceae. <u>It is thought to be both a fruit and a vegetable</u>. *Nutritional and health info:* Cantaloupe is extremely nutrient-dense, and low in calories. It is an excellent source of carotenes, potassium and other valuable nutrients, especially if the skin is juiced. It is also an excellent source of vitamins B1 (thiamine), B3 (niacin), B5 (pantothenic acid), B6 (pyridoxine), B9 (folic acid) and vitamin C (ascorbic acid) and it is a good source of dietary fiber.

Cantaloupe has been shown to contain the <u>adenosine like compound</u>. Adenosine, is an antiarrhythmic drug used to treat some forms of heart disease, relieve angina attacks (heart pain), decrease blood pressure and keep the blood thin.

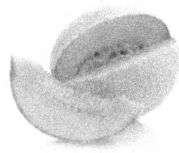

8. **Cherry** (Prunus serotina) is a small stone fruit, a drupe, which belongs to the same genus of the rose family as apricots, peaches, and plums. There are two types of cherries: sweet and sour. *Nutritional and health info*: Sour cherries are lower in calories, with 58 calories in 3 oz versus 70 calories in 3 oz of sweet cherries. Sour cherries are also higher in vitamin A, than their sweet counterparts.

In addition to their content of flavonoids, melatonin, and perillyl alcohol, both varieties of cherries contain significant amounts of several nutrients. Sour cherries are an excellent source of both vitamins A and C, and a very good source of copper and manganese. Sweet cherries are a good source of vitamin C and copper.

Cherries, like berries, are rich sources of flavonoids, specifically anthocyanidins and pro-anthocyanidins, the flavonoid molecule that give this fruit its deep red-blue color. These flavonoids exert a number of beneficial effects. They are known to inhibit cyclo-oxygenase, an enzyme produced in the body that causes inflammation and arthritic pain.

There are two forms, COX-1 cyclo-oxygenase and COX-2 cyclo-oxygenase, each of which has different purposes. The COX-1 enzyme creates prostaglandins, a hormone-like molecule that is used to send basic 'housekeeping messages to nearby cells, while the COX-2 enzyme is made in response to inflammatory processes and sends pain signal to the brain.

Most non-steroidal anti-inflammatory drugs, such as aspirin and ibuprofen, work by blocking both cyclo-oxygenase enzymes, so no pain messages are sent. Newer drugs such as Vioxx and Celebrex work by specifically blocking the COX-2 enzyme, while these drugs have been linked to serious side effects, cherries, both sour and sweet, block the COX-2 enzyme without serious side effects. Actually, researchers have found that anthocyanidins from cherries are able to block both COX-1 and COX-2 enzymes. The anthocyanidins of cherries possess antioxidant and anti-inflammatory activity superior to vitamin E.

Tart cherries have been found to contain significant quantities of melatonin, a hormone produced in the pineal gland at the base of the brain that influences the sleep process and has shown to be an effective sleep inducer.

Cherries also offer significant anti-cancer protection. Two of the anthocyanidins found in cherries – isoquerxitrin and quercetin – have been found to inhibit the growth of colon cancer. Tart cherries also contain perillyl alcohol, a natural compound that appears to be extremely powerful in reducing the incidence of all types of cancer.

Recent research suggests that perillyl alcohol shuts down the growth of cancer cells. Finally, cherries are particularly useful in the treatment of gout because they have been shown to lower the uric acid levels and prevent attacks of painful gout.

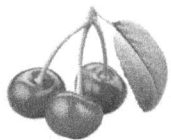

9. **Cranberry** (Vaccinium macrocarpon) is a member of the family Ericaceae, which interestingly includes rhododendrons and blueberries. *Nutritional and health info*: Raw cranberries have moderate levels of Vitamin C, dietary fiber and the essential dietary mineral, manganese, as well as a balanced profile of other essential micronutrients. Raw cranberries are a source of polyphenols antioxidants phytonutrients. These polyphenol anti-oxidant phytonutrients are presently under active

investigation for possible benefits to the cardiovascular system, immune system, and as anti-cancer agents, against prostate cancer cells.

Cranberry juice contains a material that seems to inhibit formation of plaque by Streptococcus mutans pathogens that cause tooth decay. Cranberry juice components may also decrease the formation of kidney stones.

Cranberry tannins have laboratory evidence for anti-clotting properties. Raw cranberries and unsweetened cranberry juice are abundant food sources of flavonoids such as proanthocyanidins, flavonols and quercetin. These compounds have shown possible activity as anti-cancer agents.

Cranberries are good for menopausal women as they can help prevent urinary tract infections. When you reach menopause, your body goes through changes as a result of lower estrogen levels. The reproductive and bladder tissues shrink and become less elastic and the acidity level in your vagina decreases, making you more susceptible to bladder infections and urinary tract infections (UTIs) as well as vaginal infections.

Cranberries are good for menopause as they contain proanthocyanidins, an ingredient that prevents bacteria from attaching to your bladder walls by making the bladder walls slippery.

Unsweetened cranberry juice and/or cranberry juice from concentrate are the most effective because the sugar or corn syrup in processed cranberry juice cocktails actually feed urinary infections. Cranberries are only good for prevention because once the bacteria sticks to your bladder wall you will need antibiotics to treat the infection. Your urine is usually neutral to slightly acidic, having a pH level ranging from 6 to 7. The acidic nature in your urine is what helps kill harmful bacteria. But after menopause, the acidity levels and healthy bacteria in your urine decline, allowing infectious bacteria to survive. Cranberries are also good for menopausal women because they are rich in Vitamin C and other antioxidant phytonutrients, which helps to increase the acidity level in urine.

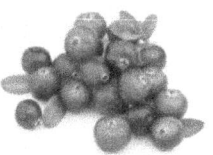

10. **Dates** (Phoenix dactylifera) grow on a date palm similar in appearance to the coconut palm. *Nutrition and health info*: Dates are an excellent source of fiber (8 grams per 3oz) and nearly all the B vitamins (B1, B2, B3, B5, B6 and B9) and the minerals: copper, potassium (200 percent more than oranges and 64 percent more than bananas), manganese, magnesium, iron, phosphorus, zinc, and selenium.

Dates are among the most alkaline (least acidic) of foods and contain a special type of soluble fiber called beta-D-glucan. This fiber has been shown to decrease the body's absorption of cholesterol and to slow or delay absorption of glucose (sugar) in the small intestine, thus helping to keep blood sugar levels even and reducing the risk of developing type 2 diabetes and heart disease.

This fiber also has the ability to absorb and hold water thus providing bulk and softness to the stools, thus easing both stool movement through the colon and elimination. This fiber can function in aiding weight loss by slowing down gastric emptying (the rate at which the stomach digests and empties its contents after a meal), thus reducing "the hunger hormone,Ghrelin" which is released by the stomach when it is empty. Therefore dates increase the feeling of satiety. Dates are also rich in anti-oxidants and anti-inflammatory nutrients. Studies indicate dates have been found to prevent free-radical damage, the main cause of all metabolic age-related medical diseases, i.e., diabetes, heart disease, hypertension, cataracts as well as certain cancers.

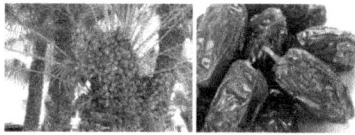

11. **Figs** (Ficus carica) are a member of the mulberry family. They have a unique sweet taste, with a chewy texture to their flesh and skin and a crunchiness to their seeds.

Nutritional and health info: Figs are high in fiber and minerals such as potassium, calcium, magnesium, iron, copper, and manganese. Figs are often recommended to nourish and tone the intestines because they are a very good source of fiber. Figs are also a good source of potassium which helps control blood pressure, maintain cardio-vascular health and support testicular health.

Also, figs are among the most highly alkaline foods and are useful in supporting the proper pH of the body. Interesting is the fact that fig leaves have anti-diabetic properties and can actually reduce the amount of insulin needed by persons with diabetes who require insulin injection.

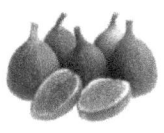

Fig leaves can also be used lower levels of triglycerides. Remember, figs resemble male testicles and are considered to have aphrodisiac properties that increases sexual desire.

12. **Grapefruit** (Citrus paradisi) belong to the rutaceae family. They are related to the orange, lemon, tangerine and pomelo. Its name comes from the fact it grows in clusters on the tree like 'grape' clusters. Also interesting, is its scientific name 'paradisi' is related the sensation of paradise because of its wonderful flavor that is juicy, tart and tangy with an underlying sweetness.

Nutritional and health info: They are very low in calories and a very good source of flavonoids, water-soluble fibers, potassium, vitamin C, and folic acid. Grapefruit also contains the phytochemicals: liminoids, flavonoids, lycopene, and glucarates. A normal serving is 3 oz serving and is equal to ½ grapefruit. This serving size contains 42 calories and 7 grams (28 calories) of fruit sugars. This serving size also contains 4 grams of fiber if you eat the inner white lining where other phytonutrients reside. Grapefruit pectin also possesses cholesterol lowering action equal to statin drugs.

Grapefruit contains excellent source of the flavonoids, **hesperidin** and **naringin. Hesperidin** is a naturally occurring bioflavonoid in citrus fruit. Hesperidin helps protect your body from conditions like hypertension, stroke and heart disease by lowering cholesterol similar to "statin" drugs and it facilitates the formation of vitamin C, which supports a healthy immune system that helps protect against most cancers.

Naringin has been shown to promote the elimination of old red blood cells by the body as well as block the cholesterol making enzyme in the liver thus reducing cholesterol levels in the blood just like the "statin" drugs do..

One interesting "tid-bit" about naringin and many other bioflavonoids is that when there is an elevation in a certain body function, this chemical will have a lowering effect, and when there is a decrease in a certain body function, it will have

41

an increasing effect. This ability of a nutrient to increase or decrease whatever is wrong is called "**modulation**".

Grapefruit appears to have this effect especially on the hematocrit and cholesterol levels. Also, grapefruit is an excellent source of the carotenoid - lycopene, which is an important phytochemical that battles heart disease, cancer and macular degeneration (a devastating eye disease).

Grapefruit is also rich in other *cancer-fighting chemicals, such as D-limonene*, which inhibits tumor formation by promoting the formation of the detoxifying enzyme **glutathione-D-transferase** in the liver.   This enzyme triggers the reaction in the liver that helps detoxify toxic compounds and make them more water-soluble so that they can be excreted from the body.

 Also, the pulp of grapefruit, contains glucarates, which are phytonutrients that may help prevent breast cancer by helping the body get rid of excess estrogen. Note- it does not interfere with normal level of estrogen – again - this a type of "**modulation.**"

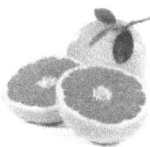

13. **Grapes** (Vitis labtrusca). Grapes are the leading fruit crop in the world. *Nutritional and health info*: Grapes provide nutritional benefits similar to those of other berries. Their nutritional quality can be enhanced by eating the seeds, which are edible in all varieties.

 Grapes are a very good source of manganese, potassium, vitamin C and the B vitamins, i.e., B1, B2, and B6. In additions to these micronutrients, grapes contain both flavonoids and the nonflavonoids.

Grapes are best known to contain the nonflavonoids, resveratrol. A 3 oz serving provides 69 calories, 15 grams (60 calories) of fruit sugars but only 1 gram of fiber. Grapes and grape seeds are excellent sources of health-promoting flavonoids. Grape seed extracts, which are rich in flavonoids known as procyanolic oligomers, are widely used in treating varicose veins.

Grapes also have the nonflavinoid resveratrol. Resveratrol acts as an anti-oxidant that is now known to reduce the buildup of cholesterol plaque in arteries: thus reducing the risk for atherosclerosis.
Remember atherosclerosis is the root cause of hypertension, stroke and heart disease. Resveratrol also has demonstrated anti-inflammatory and some anticancer action.

Grapes and grape products such as wine and grape juice, are thought to explain the "French paradox". The French eat a diet high in saturated fats and cholesterol yet have a lower risk of heart disease than Americans.

The one clue to this paradox is that the French consume a lot more grapes and red wine. Therefore, they are consuming a lot of the nonflavonoids, **resveratrol**, the anti-oxidants that protects against vascular damage, by reducing the buildup of cholesterol plaque and prevents blood platelets from clumping together, thus reducing potentially serious blood clots, heart attacks and strokes.

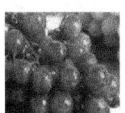

14. <u>Honeydew Melon</u> (Curcubia melo) is a member of the Cucurbitacease family. They have similar nutritional and health benefits like cucumbers and squash and cantaloupe. *Nutritional and health info:* They are an excellent source of potassium, copper, zinc and vitamin C and the B vitamins B1, B3, B5 and B6. Because of honeydew's high potassium content it is very helpful in maintaining <u>healthy blood pressure</u> levels.

Also, the nutrients (vitamin C, copper and zinc) in honeydew melon are particularly helpful for <u>healthy skin</u> and joint ligaments. These three nutrients are necessary for collagen production and tissue repair. They also contain Inositol, a very important phytonutrient, which is important in fat and cholesterol metabolism, and is a mild lipotropic agent that removes fats from the liver and lowers cholesterol.

Inositol is known to be an effective weight loss nutrient and supplement and promotes hair growth and strong healthy hair and healthy skin. Inositol is also considered <u>a brain food</u> as it works with choline for formation of lecithin, a key building block of cell membranes that protects cells from oxidation and forms the protective sheath around the brain and nerve cells.

It is an essential component of myelin that coats and regulates nerve transmission and may help prevent and treat nerve disorders, i.e., neuropathies, Parkinson's disease and Alzheimer's disease, depression and panic attacks, etc.

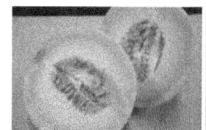 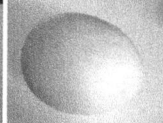

15. **Kiwifruit** (Actinidia chinensis). *Nutritional and health info*: Kiwifruit is an excellent source of the anti-oxidant vitamins A, C and E. It is also a good source of the minerals potassium, magnesium, copper, and phosphorus and a good source of fiber. One large kiwi fruit, without skin, contains 3 grams of dietary fiber per 8 grams of fruit sugar, 13 grams of carbohydrates, 56 calories, 1 gram of protein, 0 grams of fat and 0 grams of cholesterol.

   Kiwifruit is rich in anti-oxidants and enzymes which are particularly important in promoting <u>respiratory tract and digestive health</u>. Their fiber content makes kiwi fruit important for slowing down the absorption of sugars thus reducing a surge of insulin and also for removing cholesterol containing bile thus reducing the cholesterol level in the blood.

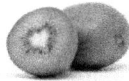

16. **Lemon / Lime** (Citrus genus) both are part of the Rutaceae family. Lemon and lime juice are mostly citric acid. Their peel consists of two layers. The outermost layer ("zest") contains essential oils that are composed mostly of limonene and citral plus a small amount of citronellal, alpha-terpineol, linalyl and geranyl acetate.

   The inner layer contains no essential oils but instead houses a variety of bitter flavones glycosides and coumarin derivatives. *Nutritional and health info*: Lemons and limes are excellent sources of vitamin C.

   In addition, they are a good source of B6 (pyridoxine) and B9 (folic acid), potassium and flavonoids and the phytonutrient limonene. A 3 oz serving contains 29 calories, 2.5 grams of fiber and only 2.5 grams of natural sugars. The phytonutrient limonene, which is extracted both lemons and limes, is showing promise in treating some cancers as well as in dissolving gallstones and kidney stones.

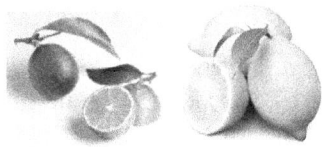

17. **Mangoes** (Mangifera indica) are a member of the sumac family (Anacardiaceae) and are a cousin to pistachios and cashew nuts. *Nutritional and health info*: Mangoes are excellent sources of carotenes, vitamin A and C, and copper, potassium and magnesium. They are also a good source of vitamins B1, B2, B3, B6, B9, and vitamin E.

The dulcet, juicy insides, of the mango - pack a nutritional punch. Its characteristic orange color is a clue to its storehouse of beta carotene (Vitamin A). Ripe mangos hold the highest levels of beta carotene, while green mangos are higher in Vitamin C.

These anti-oxidant carotenoids are known for their protective power against certain cancers. Mangos also supply ample potassium, making them ideal for hypertensive patients or anyone looking to replenish energy after physical activity. Mangoes are high in antioxidants, low in carbohydrates (although the carbohydrates are about 15% fruit sugar!)

They also contain Vitamin E and selenium which help protect against heart disease, lung disease and cancer and promote wound healing. You can obtain 40% of your daily fiber intake from a mango thus preventing constipation, piles and spastic colon. Dietary fiber also has a protective effect against degenerative diseases, especially with regards to some cancers and heart disease: such as lowering blood cholesterol levels and reducing the absorption of dietary sugar.

Mango is a good fruit for weight gain, eye disorders, hair loss, heat stroke, prickly heat, diabetes, bacterial infections, sinusitis, piles, indigestion, constipation, morning sickness, diarrhea, dysentery, scurvy, spleen enlargement, liver disorders, menstrual disorders, vaginitis, anemia and acne.

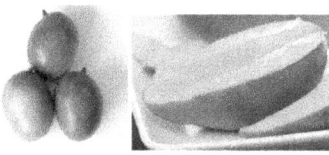

18. **Nectarines** The nectarine is a variant of peach that has a fuzzless skin. They actually belong to the same species and have arisen many times from peach trees.

Regular peach trees occasionally produce a few nectarines, and vice versa. Nectarines are more easily damaged than fuzzy peaches. Nectarines basically have the same *nutritional and health benefits* as peaches.

Just like peaches, nectarines can be white, yellow, clingstone, or freestone. They are considered a cultivar of the peach distinguished only by the absence of peach-fuzz on the skin. However, nectarines are usually sweeter than peaches.

When you eat a nectarine your body converts the carotenoid phytonutrients into vitamin A, a powerful anti-oxidant. Not only are nectarines rich in antioxidants, they are a good source of weight loss nutrients. A normal-sized nectarine will add only 50 calories to your diet, and is a good source of fiber, minerals and phytonutrients.

The orange-yellow peel of the nectarine is overflowing with phytonutrients, especially with carotenoids and flavonoids. Flavonoids are a group of phytonutrients that contain antioxidants and anti-inflammatory nutrients.

These phytonutrients help your body fight off and prevent, many cancers as well as other inflammatory chronic metabolic diseases such as heart disease (cardiovascular diseases) fibromyalgia and arthritis, diabetes, eye and kidney diseases and some of the devastating neurological disease (i.e., dementia, Alzheimer's disease and Parkinson's disease).

Anti-oxidants accomplish this by neutralizing toxins and free radicals that not only naturally accumulate as a result of metabolic processes in the body during the metabolism of glucose (oxidation) but also from environmental factors: both of which would cause damage if not neutralized.

Anti-inflammatory nutrients actually go around mending the damage done to the body's cells when free radicals, toxins and infections overwhelm the anti-oxidants.

As if that weren't enough, nectarines also provide protein and fiber. Remember, proteins are necessary for the building up of muscles and in the making of many neurotransmitters.

The fiber not only slows down the absorption of sugars and cholesterol but it also prevents constipation. Most people prefer to eat a nectarine rather than bite into a fuzzy skin peach or spend the time and trouble of peeling the skin of peaches.

Note: The pit of a nectarine as well as peaches and plums contains amygdalin, which converts to cyanide after it is eaten and digested. There is no danger in the accidental swallowing of one nectarine pit or even a habit of chewing on one or two, but eating more than that could actually result in cyanide poisoning.

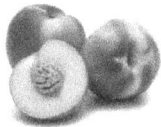

19. **Olives** (Olea europaea). Although olives are thought to be a vegetable they are technically a fruit. *Nutritional and health info*: Olives are most valued for their oil: which is oleic, an omega-9 monounsaturated fatty acid. In fact, for those of us who can remember eating oleo, oleo was really hydrogenated olive oil that is now known to be a trans-fat. Olives also are a rich source of vitamin E (tocopherols).

Olives and their oils have many unique phenolic and aromatic phytonutrients, including oleuroprein and flavonoids. The monounsaturated fats of olive oil are less likely to be involved in the production of LDL cholesterol and less likely to become oxidized than those made of other less healthy oils and saturated fats.

This is important, for as far as researchers can tell, it is only oxidized cholesterol that adheres to and invades artery walls and inevitably forms the plaque (atherosclerosis) that can lead to cardiovascular diseases (i.e., heart attacks, strokes or hypertension.

By ingesting olive oil instead of saturated animal fats, or trans-fats (hydrogenated vegetable oils) we can prevent the oxidation of cholesterol and help prevent atherosclerosis. Furthermore, when people with high cholesterol levels eliminated the saturated fat from their diet and replaced it with olive oil, total cholesterol levels dropped as well as LDL cholesterol levels dropped. However, these benefits occurred when they used olive oil instead of eating other fats, rather than simply adding olive oil to their normal diet. An important message here is the following: to reap the benefits of olive oil, the unhealthy dietary fats (especially trans-fats) still need to be eliminated from the diet. By using olive oil to cook with or use in salads other risk factors of heart disease and diabetes are lowered.

Studies have shown that those individuals who ate meals with olive oil instead or other saturated fats gained better blood sugar control, as well as lower levels of triglycerides. *(Triglycerides are another name for body fat. H*eart disease risk may also be lowered due to the anti-oxidant levels, which may protect against oxidation of cholesterol in the blood.

Also worthy of notice is that an extract found only olive leaves (Oleuropein, an anti-oxidant) can dilate the coronary arteries and helps lower blood pressure in those who are hypertensive. It also suppresses the oxidation of "LDL, the bad cholesterol molecule". Oleuropein is what give olive oil a distinctively bitter taste. Olives and olive oil may also be important in the prevention and treatment of asthma, arthritis, and cancer.

Since healthy oils are important for lowering systemic inflammation, it is not surprising that olive oil intake has also been shown to be helpful in preventing and treating arthritis and asthma symptoms. Finally, research has shown that women who regularly ingest olive oil also have a smaller risk anxiety and nervous disorders as well as breast and ovarian cancer.

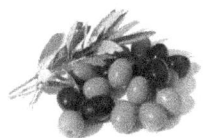

20. **Oranges** (Citrus sinensis) are in the same family as grapefruit, lemons, limes and tangerines tangelos and mandarin oranges.

   Nutritional and health info: Oranges are an excellent source of flavonoids (hesperidin) and vitamin C. They are also a good source of dietary fiber, carotenes, pectin, potassium and in B vitamins, B1 (thiamine), B2 (riboflavin), B5 (pantothenic acid), B6 (pyridoxine) and B9 (folic acid).

   Because of the high vitamin C content and flavonoids, oranges are important wherever vitamin C is required to function, especially within <u>the immune system, lens of the eye, adrenal glands, reproductive organs, in the connective tissues of our body, such as the joints, gums</u>, and in promoting overall good health.

   Like grapefruit, one of the most important flavonoids in oranges is **hesperidin.** Hesperidin has been shown to <u>lower high blood pressure as well as lower cholesterol </u>naturally, and safer than cholesterol lowering "statin" drugs.

   Hesperidin not only has anti-oxidant properties it also has strong anti-inflammatory properties which are known to repair and heal free radical damage. The inner peel and inner white pulp of the orange contains a higher concentration of hesperidin rather than in the orange flesh.

   The consumption of oranges and unprocessed orange juice has been shown to <u>protect against cancer, atherosclerosis, heart kidney and eye diseases, blood pressure, anxiety and neurological diseases </u>and <u>help fight viral infections.</u>

The pectin in oranges also possesses properties similar to that of grapefruit pectin in lowering cholesterol levels.

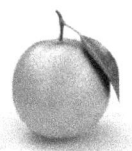

21. **Papaya** (Carica papaya). *Nutritional and health info*: Papayas are an excellent source of antioxidant nutrients, such as carotenes, vitamin C and flavonoids. They are also a very good source of folic acid, vitamins E and A, potassium, and dietary fiber. One 3 oz serving contains 2 grams of fiber to 6 grams of natural sugars.

    Papaya fruit are valued for their papain content. Papain is an enzyme that helps digest proteins. This protein-digesting enzyme is used in digestive enzyme dietary supplements. Interesting is the fact that it is also used as an ingredient in many meat tenderizers.

    In a similar manner as bromelain from pineapple it is used to treat a number of conditions, such as lung problems, indigestion, chronic diarrhea, hay fever, allergies, sports injuries and other causes of trauma. Due to papaya anti-oxidant content it also provides protective benefits against cancer, heart and eye diseases, and other diseases associated with free-radical damage.

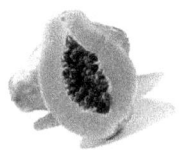

22. **Peaches** (Prunus persica). *Nutritional and health info*: Peaches and nectarines provide good levels of potassium, carotenes, flavonoids, and natural fruit sugars. Peaches and nectarines are good sources of <u>lycopene and lutein</u>, which give red, orange and yellow colors to fruits and vegetables. These phytonutrients are particularly beneficial in preventing cataracts, macular degeneration, heart disease, and cancer. See nectarines above.

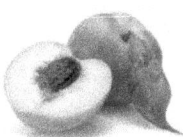

23. **Pears** (Pyrus communis). *Nutritional and health info*: Pears are a very good source of dietary fiber. They are also a good source of vitamin B2 (riboflavin), and vitamin E, and C and <u>copper</u> and potassium. A 3 oz serving that contains the skin contains 58 calories, and 5 grams of fiber to 9 grams of natural sugars. Pears are an excellent source of water-soluble fibers, including pectin. In fact, pears are actually higher in pectin than apples.

This makes them quite useful in helping to <u>lower cholesterol levels</u> and in <u>toning the intestines and preventing constipation</u>. Pears also contribute to the <u>health of skin</u> since they are high in <u>copper</u>, <u>zinc</u> and <u>vitamin C</u>. Pears are considered a hypoallergenic fruit that is high in fiber and is less likely to produce an adverse allergy response than other fruits. Particularly in the introduction of <u>fruits to infants</u>, pears are often recommended by physicians as a safe way to start fruit.

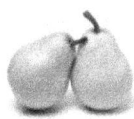

24. Pineapple (Ananas comosus). *Nutritional and health info*: Pineapples are an excellent source of vitamin C selenium and manganese, vitamin B1 (thiamine) and B6 (pyridoxine), sulfur, selenium, copper, magnesium, potassium and dietary fiber. They are free of fat and low in sodium.

They contain a sulfur containing proteolytic digestive enzymes, bromelain, that is extracted from the stem and the fruit of the pineapple that is associated with <u>preventing and healing</u> infections. While many people associate vitamin C with oranges, pineapples offer almost as much in an equivalent serving.

Vitamin C is a powerful anti-oxidant and protects against free radical damage. Remember that free radicals causes a whole host of inflammatory chronic medical diseases. The manganese in pineapples is good for <u>normal growth</u> and <u>energy production</u>.

<u>Pineapples</u> are great for reducing cardiovascular diseases, i.e., <u>blood pressure</u> and heart disease. Pineapples are the sole source of bromelain, a combination of protein-digesting enzymes and sulfur that fight inflammation in the body.

Bromelain is particularly effective in reducing inflammation associated with infection and injuries. Research indicates <u>bromelain may help treat wounds, burns, lung and sinus and throat inflammation and infections, indigestion, arthritis, and asthma</u>. However the level of bromelain in a pineapple may not be sufficient to have a medicinal effect. Bromelain tablets and capsules are available at health food stores and online.

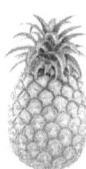

25. **Plantain:** see bananas (Musa paradisiacal) is in the same family as the banana and has the same *nutritional and health benefits* as the banana. See bananas above.

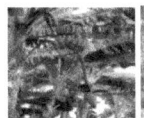 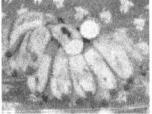

26. **Plums and prunes** (Prunus domestica) is a relative of the peach, nectarine, and almond. Like these other drupes, plums contain a hard pit or stone surrounded by soft, pulpy flesh and a thin skin. Dried plums are referred to as prunes. Prunes promote bowel regularity due to their high fiber content per serving. *Nutritional and health benefits*: see peaches and nectarines for additional info.

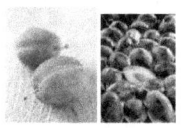

27. **Raisins** (Vitis vinifera) are the dried form of grapes. Raisins are made by dehydrating grapes. Dark brown or golden in color, raisins are naturally sweet and supply a host of vitamins and minerals.

Ancient Romans viewed raisins as a delicacy. The fruit and its beautiful vine were often used as prizes for sporting events, as money for bartering, and as decorations for places of worship.

Nutritional and health info: Raisins are a popular snack that provide many health benefits. They often appear in cookies or trail mix. Raisins are one of the fruits with the highest antioxidant content which are known to against age-related diseases such as high cholesterol, hypertension, heart disease, neurological diseases arthritis, endocrine disorders, etc. The nutrients in raisins prevent (oxidized - altered by free radicals) LDL-cholesterol from building up within artery walls. In this way raisins protect against heart disease.

One group of antioxidants in raisins, called catechins, is known to be beneficial for promoting colon health and safe and effective weight loss. There are a multitude of minerals present in a serving (1/4 cup) of raisins, as well as vitamins such as: Thiamin (B1) and Pyridoxine (B6). **Iron, calcium, potassium, boron** are the most prevalent minerals in raisins.

Raisins contain about 2g of fiber in just one 1/4-cup serving (8g of fiber in one full cup). The fiber in raisins can help relieve constipation and return bowels to normal function. A 1/4-cup of raisins also supplies about 1g of protein, making them a high-energy snack.

 The fructose and glucose content of raisins are easily absorbed by your body and converted into energy. A compound in raisins inhibits the growth of oral bacteria, which may reduce your risk of developing dental cavities and gum disease. Raisins can be used as a substitute for sodium nitrite.

Note: Sodium nitrite is often added to foods like hot dogs, bacon and lunch meats as a preservative, however, (real) sodium nitrite, the man-made preservative has been linked to cancer. Ground up raisins can preserve foods like sodium nitrite can, but without the negative side effects.

Raisins are an excellent source of the trace mineral **boron.**

Note: Boric acid has antiseptic, antifungal, and antiviral properties and for this reason is applied as a water clarifier in swimming pool water treatment. Mild solutions of boric acid have been used as eye antiseptics. Some boron compounds show promise in treating arthritis.

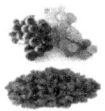

28. **Raspberries** (Rubus idseus) are related to blackberries and have basically the same _nutritional and health benefits_.

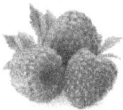

29. **Strawberries** (Fragaria) are the most popular type of berry in the world. _Nutritional and health info_: Strawberries are an excellent source of vitamin C and K, dietary fiber and flavonoids. They are also a good source of vitamin B1, B5, B6, B7 and B9, manganese, magnesium, copper, iron and iodine. A 3 oz serving contains 32 calories and 3 grams fiber and 4 grams of fruit sugars.

The health benefits of strawberries are due primarily to their flavonoid phytonutrients (anthocyanidin -pelargonidin) and vitamin C. Sliced strawberries also provide 40 mcg of folic acid (B9) per cup, which helps protect the health of your red blood cells and protects fetuses from developing specific birth defects as well as protects against memory problems as we age.

Also, one cup has 254 mg of potassium, a fluid-balancing mineral that also reduces blood pressure. The antioxidants in strawberries can also play a role in lowering cholesterol due to their high fiber content. Also because strawberries are high in iodine they are useful for <u>improving thyroid function</u>.

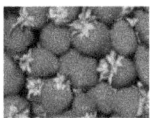

30. **<u>Tangerines</u>** belong to the same family of citrus fruits as oranges and basically have the same *nutritional and health benefits* as oranges. <u>See oranges above.</u>

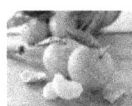

31. **<u>Watermelon</u>** (Citrullus lanatus) is a member of the Cucurbitaceae family, along with cantaloupe, squash, pumpkin and other plants that grow on vines on the ground.

Nutritional and health info: Watermelon is very low in calories with one cup containing only 48 calories, yet it is still a good source of <u>vitamin A, B1, B5, B6, B7 and C, beta-carotene, and Lycopene, magnesium, potassium</u> and dietary <u>fiber</u>.

 Watermelon is an <u>excellent diuretic</u>. It is a good source of many minerals but its most prominent mineral is potassium. Potassium is a positively charged electrolyte important for the healthy functioning of <u>blood pressure, heart, kidneys, muscles, nerves</u>.

Watermelon also contains <u>phosphorus, magnesium, calcium</u>. Phosphorus is essential for the formation of your bones and teeth and the synthesis of protein for the growth, maintenance and repair of your tissues and to make ATP, the energy molecule in your body.

Magnesium is important for your bone structure and strength, muscle relaxation, heart rhythm, nerve conductance, immunity, metabolism and blood glucose regulation.

Calcium is important for bone health, as well as crucial for nerve transmission and contraction of both skeletal and cardiac muscle. Other minerals in watermelon include small amounts of sodium, iron, selenium, manganese, copper, zinc.

Watermelon helps combat fatigue and boosts energy levels. Lycopene is known for its anti-cancer capability. Watermelon is high in arginine. Arginine reduces stress, anxiety, and panic attacks, kidney stones as well as treats erectile dysfunction in men. Arginine also plays a role in reducing blood pressure because it relaxes the muscles in blood vessels.

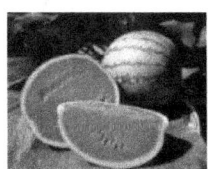

CHAPTER 4   VEGETABLES AND THEIR HEALTH BENEFITS

Vegetables have a long history of providing nutrients that are known to prevent and/or heal many metabolic medical diseases. These modern-day inflammatory metabolic diseases are type 2 diabetes: cardiovascular diseases such as hypertension, high cholesterol, high triglycerides, Heart attack i.e., myocardial Infarctions (MI) and strokes (CVA): many nervous systems diseases, dementia, Alzheimer's disease, even anxiety and depression: kidney and eye diseases: arthritis: fibromyalgia and even most cancers.

These diseases are mainly due to deficiencies of both inflammatory and anti-oxidant phytonutrients, minerals and vitamins that are naturally found in vegetables. More and more evidence is accumulating showing that vegetables can prevent, as well as treat, many of these modern day medical diseases, especially chronic degenerative diseases mentioned above.

 Vegetables provide the broadest range of nutrients and phytochemicals, especially fiber and carotene phytonutrients, of any food class. They are also rich sources of carbohydrates, and protein, and the little fat they contain is in the form of essential fatty acids, such as the omega-3, and omega-6. Vegetables should play a major role in your diet. We should consume a minimum of three to five servings of vegetables per day.

1. **Arugula** is a powerfully cruciferous, mustard like green leafy vegetable used mostly in salads. *Nutritional health info*: Arugula contains manganese, magnesium, potassium,

calcium, copper, iron, zinc and it is an excellent source of Vitamins: A, B2 (riboflavin), B7 (folic acid) and "C", as well as powerful anti-oxidant phyto-nutrients such as: carotenes and chlorophyll. Arugula contains a group of **anti-cancer compounds** known as glucosinolates that are potent antioxidants and stimulators of natural detoxifying enzymes (i.e., **glutathione S-transferase** and **glucuronyl transferases**) in the body. Juices and extracts of these vegetable are good for helping the liver and blood to detoxify foreign, toxic substances and prevent disease.

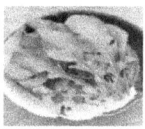

2. **Asparagus** is a member of the lily family. It is prized for its nutritional food value and for its medicinal properties.

Nutritional and health info: It is low in carbohydrates and calories and at the same time is rich in protein as well as potassium, phosphorus, iron, and vitamins: A, C, K, and B1 (thiamine), B2 (riboflavin), B3 (niacin, B6 (pyridoxine), B7 (folic acid). It is also a good source of dietary fiber.

Nutrients in asparagus are used to treat arthritis due to a unique phytonutrients, (**racemofuran** and **asparagamine**). These phytonutrients are inhibitors of the COX-2 enzyme. Asparagus also has nutrients that act as a diuretic due to the amino acid **asparagine**.

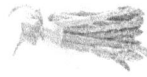

3.   **Beets** (Beta vulgaris) belong to the same family as chard and spinach (Chenopodiaceae). However, unlike these greens, both the root and the leaves of beets are eaten.
Nutrition and health info: The root has a high sugar and fiber content, and is delicious when eaten raw but is more typically cooked or pickled. Beets are the main ingredient in *borscht*, a traditional eastern European soup.

Beet greens are rich in calcium, iron, manganese, potassium and Vitamins A and C. Beet roots are excellent source of folic acid and fiber. Both greens and root are a good source of magnesium, phosphorus, iron and vitamin B6 (pyridoxine). Beets have long been used for medicinal purposes, primarily for disorders of the liver, given their stimulating effects on the liver's detoxification processes and for their anti-cancer properties.

The pigment that gives beets their rich, purple-crimson color, betacyanin, is a powerful cancer-fighting agent. Beet fiber has been shown to have a favorable effect on bowel function and cholesterol levels too.

Beet fiber has been shown to increase the level of the detoxifying enzymes, specifically glutathione peroxidase and glutathione-S-transferase.

It also increases the number of special white blood cells responsible for detecting and eliminating abnormal cells. Beet juice has been found to be a potent inhibitor of the formation of nitrosamines (cancer-causing compounds derived primarily from the ingestion of nitrates from smoke or cured meats as well as the cell mutations caused by these compounds.

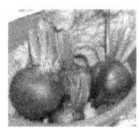

4. **Bell Peppers** (Capsicum annuum) is a member of the Solanaceae or nightshade family, which includes potatoes, eggplants, and tomatoes. They are available in several colors: green peppers have a slightly bitter flavor, while red, orange, and yellow peppers are sweeter flavor.

    Nutritional and health info: The spices pimento and paprika are both prepared from red bell peppers. They exert a protective effect against cataracts, due to their vitamin C and beta-carotene content and many different powerful phytonutrients: such as the phenol (capsaicin) & the flavonoids (quercetin, catechin, and flavones) that prevent blood clot formation, reduce the risk of heart attacks, lower cholesterol and blood pressure naturally, prevent some cancers, and decrease muscle and joint pain.

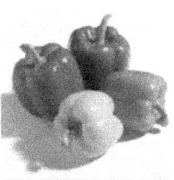

5. **Bitter Melon** or **Balsam Pear** (Momordica charantia) is a green cucumber-shaped gourd-like vegetable with bumps all over it. It is in the same family, Cucurbitaceae, with squash and watermelon. The fruit of the bitter melon is also known as the balsam pear.

    Nutritional and Health info: Bitter melon can be prepared as an herbal remedy in many ways and used for treating diverse health problems. Bitter melon can be used to treat stomach problems, respiratory problems, skin breakages, headaches and blood sugar issues. Bitter melon leaves and seeds are ground into a juice that is imbibed to cure parasites, diarrhea and other stomach issues, as well as coughs and respiratory infections. Warm leaves are applied to skin to treat burns or cuts. For other ailments, such as headaches or blood sugar problems as well as detoxification drinking juice from the fruit and leaves is best.

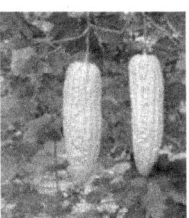

6. **Broccoli** is a member of the cruciferous or cabbage family. *Nutritional and Health info*: Broccoli is low in calories and is one of the most nutrient-dense foods. It is especially rich in vitamin A, C, E, and K as well as pyridoxine (B6), folic acid (B9), and fiber. It is also a very good source of phosphorus, potassium and magnesium . It is an excellent source of protein and fiber. Broccoli also contains phytonutrients such as glucosinolates, sulforaphane and the carotenoid, lutein.

Broccoli, like other members of the cabbage family demonstrates remarkable anti-cancer effects, particularly in breast and gastric cancer. Sulforaphane has also proven to be effective in helping the body get rid of Helicobacter pylori, a bacterium that is responsible for most peptic ulcers and also increases a person's risk of getting gastric cancer.

This bacterium is also linked to causing a wide range of other stomach disorders, including gastritis, esophagitis, and acid indigestion. In fact, broccoli contains the highest concentration of protective nutrients. These protective nutrients have been found to even reduce the size of cancerous tumors.

These nutrients stimulate the body's production of detoxification enzymes and exert anti-oxidant effects throughout the body. Indole-3-carbinol is also an important cancer-fighting phytonutrient, as it has been shown to arrest growth of both breast and prostate cancer cells in preliminary studies.

These phytonutrients also increase the ability of the liver to detoxify toxic compounds as well as decreases the growth of the human papilloma virus (a virus linked to cervical cancer). Broccoli is also a rich source of lutein. Lutein is a carotenoid phytonutrient that has anti-cancer properties and is helpful in preventing cataracts and the development of age-related macular degeneration. Lutein acts to protect the retina from damage.

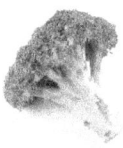

7. **Brussels Sprouts** are developed from the wild cabbage. They resemble miniature cabbages and basically have the same *nutritional and health benefits* as cabbage. See cabbage below.

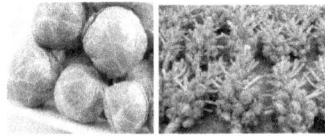

8. **Cabbage** belongs to the cruciferous family of vegetables. This family also includes broccoli, Brussels sprouts,

cauliflower, collards, kale, mustard greens, radishes, rutabaga, and turnips. *Nutritional and Health info*: Cabbage is a nutrient-dense, low-calorie food providing an excellent source of many nutrients, especially vitamins C, B6 (pyridoxine), B7 (biotin), B9 (folic acid), potassium, calcium, magnesium and manganese.

But more importantly than the vitamin and mineral content of cabbage is its phytonutrient content. In particular, cabbage like broccoli contains the powerful anti-cancer phytonutrients known as glucosinolates. Including cruciferous vegetables, such as cabbage, broccoli, Brussels sprouts, and cauliflower, in the diet on a regular basis is known to reduce the risk of cancer.

This is because the cabbage family of vegetables contains more phytonutrients with anti-cancer properties than any other vegetable family. Most of these phytonutrients are glucosinolates, a phytonutrient in the indole class along with sulforaphane, indole-3-carbinol, di-indolmethane, and isothiocyanates.

Consistently, the higher the intake of cabbage-family vegetables, the lower the rates of cancer, particularly colon, prostate, lung, and breast cancer. The glucosinolates in cabbage work primarily by increasing anti-oxidant defense mechanisms and improving the body's ability to detoxify and eliminate harmful chemicals and hormones.

Another anti-cancer component of cabbage was identified as the amino acid, glutamine. Glutamine is a critical factor in the growth and regeneration of the cells that line the gastrointestinal tract. Also, cabbage has been shown to be extremely effective in the treatment of peptic ulcers.

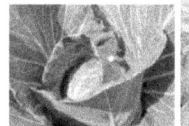 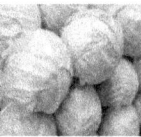

9. **Carrots** (Daucus carota. Carrots belong to the Umbelliferae family, which include parsnips, parsley, fennel, and dill. *Nutritional and Health info*: The carrot provides the highest source of pro-vitamin A carotenes of the commonly consumed vegetables.

They also provide excellent levels of vitamin K, B7 (biotin) and fiber and very good levels of vitamin C, B1 (thiamine), B6 (pyridoxine), and potassium. One 3oz serving provides 41 calories with 9 grams of carbohydrate as 4 grams of fruit sugar (fructose and glucose) and 3 grams of fiber.

 Carrots are an excellent source of carotenoid-rich foods that provide antioxidant phytonutrients. These phytonutrients help protect against cardiovascular disease and some cancers. High carotene intake has been linked with a decrease in post-menopausal breast cancer and a decrease in the incidence of cancers of the bladder, cervix, prostate, colon, larynx, lung and esophagus.

Carrots also promote good vision, especially night vision. In fact, beta-carotene, along with other carotenoids, lutein and zeaxanthin, which are present in high quantities in carrots, provide protection against macular degeneration and the development of senile cataracts, the leading cause of blindness in the elderly.

Carotenes are stored in adipose tissue, the liver, the adrenals, testes, and ovaries and skin. Ingesting large quantities of carotenes can lead to a yellowing of the skin known as carotenodermia. This occurrence is not serious: in fact, it may be beneficial in protecting against sun damage to the skin.

Sometimes this condition, carotenodermia, is not directly attributable to dietary intake or supplementation, as it may be indicative of a deficiency in a necessary factor in the conversion of beta-carotene to vitamin "A", such as deficiencies of zinc, thyroid hormone, vitamin C, and dietary protein.

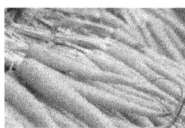

10. **Cauliflower** is a member of the cruciferous vegetable family, which includes broccoli, kale and cabbage. Cauliflower is not as nutrient dense as the many other cabbage family vegetables, but it is still power packed with nutrition.

    Nutritional and Health info: Raw cauliflower is an excellent source of vitamin K and C and is a very good source of fiber, boron, potassium, phosphorus, and all the B vitamins. Its white color is a sign that it has much less of the beneficial carotenes and chlorophyll found in other cruciferous vegetables: however, cauliflower along with beets broccoli, nuts, grapes, prunes, raisins, apples, pears oranges, avocadoes, peas, carrots, and beans is a good source of the mineral boron.

    Cauliflower contains phytonutrients that may help prevent cancer. These compounds increase the activity of detoxifying enzymes that disable and eliminate toxic carcinogens and other free radicals.

 The mineral <u>boron</u> is known to increase levels of both <u>estrogen and testosterone thus increasing sex drive and reducing hot flashes</u>. Boron also decreases inflammation and therefore the pain of arthritis and inflamed muscles and ligaments. Boron also plays a role in treating depression, mental fatigue and memory loss. <u>Note: Boron poor soil can be treated with Borax.</u>

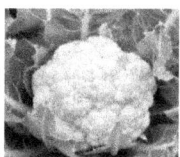

11. **Celery** is a member of the Umbelliferae family, along with carrots, parsley and fennel. It is a biennial vegetable, meaning it has a normal growing cycle of once every two years. While most people associate celery with its stalks, its leaves, roots, and seeds are also used as food and seasoning.

 Nutritional and Health info: Celery is an excellent source of vitamin C and fiber. It is also a good source of potassium, vitamin B1 (thiamine), B6 (pyridoxine), and B9 (folic acid). While celery contains more sodium than most other vegetables, the sodium is offset by a very high level of potassium. Celery is known to be good for sustaining strong bones.

Celery contains phytonutrients known as <u>coumarins</u>, which are shown to be useful in <u>cancer prevention</u> and treatments as they are capable of enhancing the activity of certain white blood cells. The phytonutrient <u>Coumarin</u> also tones the vascular system, lowers blood pressure, lowers cholesterol and may be useful in cases of migraine headache.

Celery produces a diuretic effect (much like watermelon) thereby lowering blood pressure. Celery juice is a great electrolyte replacement drink, especially after workouts and is useful in detoxification.

Celery seed extract has been shown to produce significant benefits in the treatment of both acute and chronic 'rheumatism' pain. Rheumatism is the general term for arthritis and muscular problems. This extract also lowers the production of uric acid by inhibiting the enzyme xanthine oxidase and thus prevents gout. Gout is a very painful arthritic condition where uric acid crystals build up within joints.

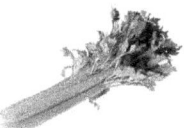

12. **Chard,** (Swiss chard).belong the Amaranthaceae and the subfamily Betoideae. Chard belongs to the same family as beets and spinach and it shares a similar taste profile: that is, the bitterness of beet greens and the slightly salty flavor of spinach leaves. Chard has been bred to have highly nutritious leaves at the expense of the root (which is not as nutritious as the leaves).

Chard leaves (greens) is considered to be one of the healthiest vegetables available and a valuable addition to a healthy diet (like other green leafy vegetables). Swiss chard, along with kale, mustard greens and collard greens, is one of several leafy green vegetables often referred to as "**greens**". It is a tall leafy green vegetable with a thick, crunchy stalk that comes in white, red or yellow with wide fan-like green leaves. Both the leaves and stalk of chard are edible, although the stems vary in texture with the white ones being the most tender.

Nutritional and Health Benefits-Swiss chard has concentrations of vitamins A, C, E, K, B1 (thiamine), B2 (riboflavin), B3 (niacin), B5 (pantothenic acid), B6 (pyridoxine), B7 (folate), copper, calcium, phosphorous, zinc, magnesium, manganese, potassium, iron, protein, dietary fiber and many phytonutrients such as choline, inositol, kaempferol, isorhamnetin, coumestans,and oxalic acid to mention a few. Swiss chard is important for maintaining bone health.

One cup of Swiss chard contains just 35 calories, but provides 109.9% of the daily value for vitamin A. Both vitamin A and beta-carotene are important vision nutrients. Beta-carotene has also been the subject of extensive research in relationship to cancer prevention and prevention of oxygen-based (oxidation) damage to cells.

Beta-carotene may help to protect against certain forms of cancer since it belongs to the family known as carotenoids. Magnesium, helps regulate nerve and muscle tone by balancing the action of calcium.

 In many nerve cells, **magnesium serves as nature's own calcium channel blocker**, preventing calcium from rushing into the nerve cell and activating the nerve.

By blocking calcium's entry, magnesium keeps our nerves and the blood vessels and muscles they enervate relaxed thus reducing blood pressure like prescription "calcium channel blockers" (i.e., verapamil, diltiazem, amlodipine). Magnesium, as well as calcium, is necessary for healthy bones.

About two-thirds of the magnesium in the human body is found in our bones. Some magnesium helps give bones their physical structure, while the rest is found on the surface of the bone where it is stored for the body to draw upon as needed.

Swiss chard can promote your cardiovascular health by being an excellent source of not only magnesium but also potassium. Potassium is an important electrolyte found in chard. Potassium is involved in nerve transmission and the contraction of all muscles including the heart. Potassium is essential for maintaining normal blood pressure and heart function.

Swiss chard an especially good choice to prevent high blood pressure and protect against atherosclerosis. Swiss chard is an excellent source of vitamin C. Vitamin C can neutralize free radicals and it can help prevent the oxidation of LDL-cholesterol. (*i.e., oxidized LDL-cholesterol is the bad alteration of LDL-cholesterol. Note, recent studies indicate that it is only the oxidized LDL-cholesterol that can damage the inner lining of artery walls. Free radicals oxidize LDL-cholesterol. Only after being oxidized does LDL-cholesterol stick to artery walls, building up in plaques.*)

Vitamin C, which is also vital for the proper function of a healthy immune system, is good for preventing colds and may be helpful in preventing recurrent ear infections. Swiss chard is an excellent source of iron, a mineral so vital to the health of the human body.

Iron is primarily linked with protein to form the oxygen-carrying molecule hemoglobin, which is why insufficient iron can quickly translate into anemia. Iron enhances oxygen distribution throughout your body, keeps your immune system healthy and helps your body produce energy. Swiss chard is an excellent source of <u>vitamin E, the body's primary fat-soluble antioxidant</u>.

Anti-inflammatory and cardiovascular benefits from Swiss chard are also due to is containing a good source of Vitamin E. Vitamin E travels throughout the body neutralizing free radicals that would otherwise damage fat-containing structures and molecules, such as cell membranes, brain cells, and cholesterol.

By protecting these cellular and molecular components, vitamin E has significant anti-inflammatory effects that result in the reduction of symptoms in <u>hypertension</u>, heart disease, <u>asthma, osteoarthritis, and rheumatoid arthritis</u>, some eye, kidney, and neurological disease and some cancerous conditions where free radicals and inflammation play a big role. Vitamin E has also been shown to reduce the risk of colon cancer, help decrease the severity and frequency of hot flashes in women going through menopause, and help reduce the development of diabetes.

Swiss chard's health benefits continue with its fiber: a cup of Swiss chard provides 14.7% of the daily value for fiber, which has been shown to reduce blood sugar levels and high cholesterol levels thus helping to prevent atherosclerosis and other related diseases.

Because fiber can also help out by keeping blood sugar levels under control, Swiss chard is an excellent vegetable for people with diabetes. Swiss chard's fiber also binds to cancer-causing chemicals, keeping them away from the cells lining.

All parts of the chard plant contain oxalic acid. Chard has a slightly bitter taste and is used in a variety of cultures around the world, including Arab cuisine.

Fresh young chard can be used raw in salads. Mature chard leaves and stalks are typically cooked (like in sautéed): their bitterness fades with cooking, leaving a refined flavor which is more delicate than that of cooked spinach.

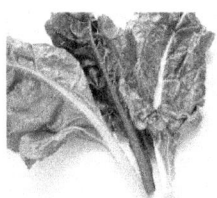

13. **Chili Pepper.** Chili peppers are used to make Cayenne (Red) Pepper. They are members of the nightshade family, Solanaceae. They not only add a lot of flavor to our food but they also have a wide range of health benefits as well. Chilies produce capsaicin, a medicinal phytonutrient: this is what produces the hot burning sensation we feel in our mouth. Beyond leaving our mouth on fire, chili peppers have health benefits as well.

Nutritional and Health info: Scientists have proven that capsaicin can reduce cancer cells. There have been several scientific clinical studies completed that have shown that natural capsaicin directly slows and reduces the growth of leukemic cells.

Capsaicin is a natural antioxidant and helps protect against disease caused by toxins and free radicals. Capsaicin is an active ingredient in many of the most popular "fat burning" supplements on the market. A thermogenic agent, capsaicin helps to increase overall the metabolism rate and helps the body burn calories and unwanted fat deposits.

Peppers are a natural anti-inflammatory. They can help prevent and relieve arthritis. Eating hot chili peppers helps maintain strong cell walls in your circulatory system and will help lower your blood pressure naturally.

 People who suffer from cluster headaches and migraines can rub chili peppers on the temples to find relief. Capsicum increases endorphins and other mood elevating, good feeling chemicals, thus, it helps fight depression, reduces pain and relieves stress.

 Hot chilies slow down the growth of H. pylori, the bacteria that causes certain kinds of ulcers.   Psoriasis and other skin conditions benefit from spicy foods and can help heal the skin.

Chilies have been shown to have a positive effect on an overactive bladder by blocking contractions that cause unpredictable loss of urine. Spicy foods will help increase sex drive and libido and will improve your love life. A good bowl of hot chili is always a great meal on a cold winter day. Not only does it warm us up, it also helps protect us from common winter colds and lung infections.

Capsicum can reduce cold/flu symptoms, sinusitis, and respiratory problems. It is a natural remedy for herpes. Cut a chili pepper open and rub it and watch the infection disappear.

Capsicum ointment is now available in the form of a prescription drug. It can be applied directly to the skin to aid in healing and controlling the pain associated with herpes.

Capsicum is a natural muscle relaxant and pain reliever. There are also a number of creams that have capsicum in them to soothe and heal painful muscles. Capsaicin is a safe and effective topical analgesic agent in the management of arthritis pain, herpes zoster-related pain, diabetic neuropathy, post mastectomy pain, and headache.

When consumed, capsaicinoid phytonutrients bind to pain receptors in the mouth and throat that are responsible for sensing heat. Once activated by the capsaicinoids, these receptors send a message to the brain that the person has consumed something hot. The brain responds to the burning sensation by raising the heart rate, increasing perspiration and releasing endorphins (natural endogenous opiates). Endorphins are considered to be endogenous opioid peptides that function as neurotransmitters.

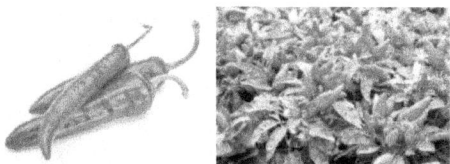

14. **Collards,** (Brassica oleradea). Collard (also known as tree-cabbage or non-heading cabbage), is a cool-season vegetable green that is rich in vitamins and minerals. It can be grown in warm weather and can tolerate more cold weather in the late fall than any other member of the cabbage family.

Brassica oleracea are part of the Acephala Group of vegetables which contains cabbage and broccoli. Collards are a popular substitute for cabbage in the Deep South. They are fibrous, tough, mild-flavored greens that require long cooking.

Nutritional and Health info: Collards are a good source of iron and ascorbic acid (vitamin C). Collards present an interesting, flavorful, and nutritious alternative to dishes that call for cabbage, kale or a similar type of vegetable.

They are an excellent source of beta carotene and some vitamin C and Calcium. The darker the leaf the more beta carotene it contains.

Like broccoli, kale and cabbage, the antioxidants and phytonutrients in collards may help to reduce the risk of some forms of cancer and heart disease.

Note: you can combine collards with black-eyed peas as a side dish: you can also chop cooked collards and add them as an ingredient to stuffing or, sautéing them with ham, garlic, and onions to serve as an entrée. They contain no fat or cholesterol and are low in sodium and calories.

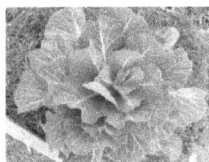

15. **Corn** is a very unusual vegetable. Corn also known as sweet corn or maize, is not only delicious but also stuffed with nutrients and high in fiber.

Nutritional and Health benefits: Corn provides the phytonutrients, lutein and zeaxanthin. Both of these phytonutrients are considered carotenoids and are known to prevent and treat eye diseases.

Lutein and zeaxanthin usually are found together and both these carotenoids are essential nutrients to avoid the risk of eye degeneration. Zeaxanthin is the yellow pigment and is essential to protect the retina from damaging effects of light.

The Health _benefits_ of corn include: fighting against free radicals thus reducing the risk of certain serious lung problems and reducing the risk of some cancers. Corn contains the powerful antioxidants beta carotene, and beta cryptoxanthin.

Beta cryptoxanthin may reduce the risk of developing inflammatory disorders such as rheumatoid arthritis. Corn is also an excellent source of vitamin A, which is known for its positive effect on vision. Vitamin A may also aid in building your immune function, bone metabolism and skin health.

One of the other health benefits of corn is in the contents of the B vitamins especially folate. Folate(B9) may reduce the risk of Alzheimer's disease and reduce neural tube defect which are defects affecting the brain and spinal cord. Women who are capable of getting pregnant should take adequate amount of folate.

Corn contains dietary fiber which is useful for colon health. The potassium present in corn will benefit your heart, muscles and kidney function. And phosphorus corn contains is necessary to help develop strong bones and teeth, remove toxins through the kidney and provides the body with energy (ATP).

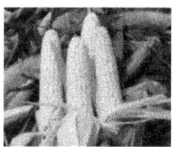

16. **Cucumbers** (Cucumis sativus) are in the vine growing Cucurbitaceae family. This family of vegetables also includes: watermelon, gherkins, cantaloupe, honeydew melons, muskmelon, squash and pumpkins.

 Nutrition and Health info: Cucumbers are composed primarily of water but still pack a lot of nutritional value. The flesh of cucumbers is a very good source of vitamins A, C and B9 (folic acid).

The hard skin is rich in fiber and contains a variety of important minerals, including silica, potassium, magnesium, and molybdenum. A 3 oz serving provides only 12 calories as carbohydrates. Cucumber is an excellent source of silica, a trace mineral that contributes to the strength of our connective tissue. It is the intracellular cement, muscles, tendons, ligaments, cartilage, and bone.

Cucumbers are also used topically for various types of skin problems, including swelling under the eyes and sunburn. Two nutrients in cucumbers, ascorbic acid (vitamin C) and caffeic acid, help reduce swelling.

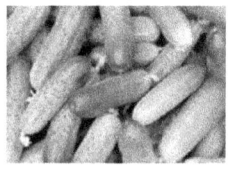

17. **Dandelions** belong to the sunflower (Compositae) family
    and the Taraxacum genus. Vegetables in this genus have
    the ability to correct a multitude of disorders. Dandelions
    are perennial plants that are both a weed and a vegetable.

    Nutritional and Health info: One cup of dandelions contains
    only 25 calories, yet it is exceptionally high in nutrient. It is
    particularly high in vitamins and minerals, protein, the
    pectin fiber and phytonutrients such as choline and inulin.
    Dandelions are an excellent source of vitamin A, C, B1
    (thiamine), B2 (riboflavin), B6 (pyridoxine), calcium, copper,
    manganese, and iron.

    Dandelions are a rich source of nutrients and other
    compounds that (1) detoxify the blood and liver, (2)
    improve liver functions, (3) promote weight loss, (4) possess
    diuretic activity, and (5) improve blood sugar control.

    Dandelion root is especially good for the health of the liver.
    Dandelion extract has been shown to improve the
    production of liver enzymes that act as anti-oxidants. They
    enhance the flow of bile.

    Nutrients in dandelion roots can prevent and treat
    conditions such as liver congestion, bile duct inflammation,
    hepatitis, gallstones, and jaundice. Nutrients in dandelion
    are being used as a weight loss aid in the treatment of
    obesity.

    Research has also revealed that dandelion root contains a
    very high concentration of an indigestible carbohydrate
    called inulin, which serves as a food source for friendly
    colonic bacteria, i.e., *Bifidobacterium* and *Lactgovacillus*.

When these beneficial bacteria are encouraged to proliferate, they crowd out other harmful bacteria thus acting like a natural, selective, protective antibiotic and improving the health of the digestive tract.   Inulin is also helpful in improving blood sugar control (improves diabetic control).   Inulin in dandelions is known to decrease blood sugar, LDL-cholesterol and triglyceride levels as well as raise levels of beneficial HDL-cholesterol.

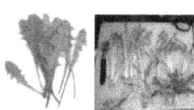

18. **Egg Plant** (Solanum melongena) belongs to the nightshade plant family (Solanaceae) along with the tomato and potato. *Nutritional and Health info*: Eggplant is an excellent source of dietary fiber. It is also a very good source of vitamins B1 (thiamine) and B6 (pyridoxine) and potassium, copper, magnesium, manganese, phosphorus, (B3) niacin, and folic acid (B9). Eggplant contains an anthocyanin flavonoid called nasunin. Nasunin is a potent antioxidant and free-radical scavenger that protects cell membranes from damage. Nasunin protects the lipids (fats) from becoming oxidized in brain cell membranes.

Cell membranes are almost entirely composed of lipids and are responsible for protecting the cell from free radicals, as well as responsible for letting nutrients in and wastes out, and receiving instructions from messenger molecules that tell the cell which activities it should perform.

 Nasunin is not only a potent free radical scavenger, but it also helps remove excess iron out of the body. Although iron is an essential nutrient too much iron is not a good thing. Excess iron increases free-radical production and is associated with an increase risk of heart disease and cancer.

Menstruating women, who lose iron every month in their menstrual flow, are unlikely to be at risk, but in post-menopausal women and men, iron, which is not easily excreted, can accumulate.

By helping to bind excess iron, nasunin lessens free-radical production with numerous beneficial results, including protecting blood LDL-cholesterol from becoming oxidized LDL-cholesterol, the toxic form that damages the inner lining of the artery walls.

By reducing free-radical production, nasunin can prevent cellular damage that could promote or trigger cancer cells. It also lessens free-radical damage in joints, a primary factor in arthritis. Eggplant also has been found to lower cholesterol, relax arterial wall muscle and reduce high blood pressure.

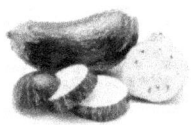

19. **Endive** belongs to the chicory family of greens. _Nutritional info_: each leaf contains only <u>one calorie</u>. It is an excellent source of vitamin A and C, carotenes and fiber. _Health info_: It has been shown to help <u>insomnia</u> and in <u>purifying the blood</u>.

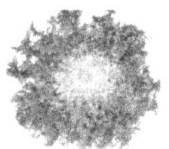 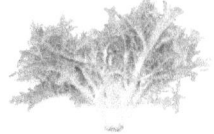

20. **Fennel** (Foeniculum vulgare) is a member of the Umbelliferae family along with carrots, celery and parsley. It is known as a vegetable and an herb. Nutritional and Health info: The bulbs, stalks, leaves and seeds are all edible. Fennel has a long history of use as a medicinal plant. (1) An intestinal antispasmodic, (2) a carmi-native or compound that relieves or expels gas.

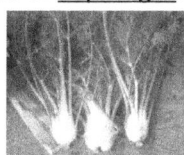

21. **Garlic** (Allium sativum) is a member of the lily family. *Nutritional and Health info*: Garlic is an excellent source of vitamin A, B6, and C as well as a good source of manganese, selenium, phosphorus, calcium, potassium, sulfur, iron and copper. One 3 oz serving provides 150 calories with 6 grams being protein and 2 grams of fiber.

 Most of garlic's therapeutic properties are thought to be due to its sulfur containing compounds, allicin, diallyl disuldide, diallyl trisulfide. Sulfur can be used as an antibiotic and is in several prescription medications including Celebrex.

Garlic has a long history of being used as an infection fighter. In fact in Russia, it is referred to as "Russian Penicillin" because of it anti-bacterial properties. The antimicrobial activity is due to allicin. Allicin has been shown to be effective against the common cold, and flu, stomach viruses and yeast infection.

Garlic appears to provide protection against atherosclerosis, heart disease, diabetes, asthma, and some gastrointestinal problems. Many studies have shown that garlic decreases total serum cholesterol levels while increasing serum HDL cholesterol levels. HDL cholesterol seems to have a protective factor against heart disease.

Garlic has also demonstrated blood pressure – lowering action in many studies. Garlic also appears to offer protection against some cancers, especially colon cancer.

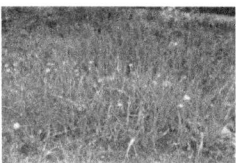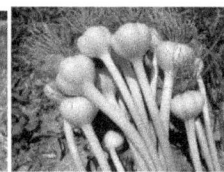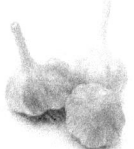

22. **Jerusalem Artichoke** The Jerusalem artichoke (Helianthus tuberosus), also called sunroot, sunchoke, earth apple or topinambour, is a species of sunflower It is an edible tuber or underground stem of a native American plant belonging to the sunflower family (Asteraceae). Jerusalem artichokes are not related to the domestic artichoke.

The Jerusalem artichoke is considered both a food and a medicinal vegetable. It can grow to heights of 5-10 feet and look much like sunflowers in the field. They have upright hearty yellow flowers 2-3 inches in diameter, 4-8 inch long hairy leaves and thick, hairy stems.

It can grow domesticated in fields or wild along streams . The edible part is the tuber or under-ground stem (root). Jerusalem Artichoke tubers can be eaten raw, boiled or baked like potatoes.

The Jerusalem Artichoke looks like a knobby, odd-shaped root similar to a ginger root. The firm, crisp tubers are low in starch and taste a bit like water chestnuts, i.e., a sweet nutty flavor.

Nutritional and Health Info: One cup of Jerusalem artichokes contains 109 calories. Jerusalem artichokes are a good source of fiber, inulin, thiamine, phosphorus, potassium and iron. They are low in saturated fat, cholesterol and sodium.

Jerusalem artichokes are considered a valuable food or dietary supplement for people suffering from diabetes and other pancreatic complaints because it is known to reduce blood sugar levels and minimize the need for insulin.

Unlike the potato where its starch breaks down to glucose affecting blood sugar, the Jerusalem Artichoke is high in inulin which only breaks down to fructose in the colon.

As a result, they are considered to have a very low glycemic index and Inulin, the carbohydrate found in Jerusalem artichokes, is counted as a pro-biotic because it is not readily digestible. (Inulin is different from insulin but perhaps mimics it).

Inulin can prevent and/or help with the relief constipation. It not only lowers blood glucose levels, but it also improves calcium absorption, the reduction of triglycerides and LDL cholesterol blood levels. Inulin is also known to inhibit the growth of various kinds of cancer.

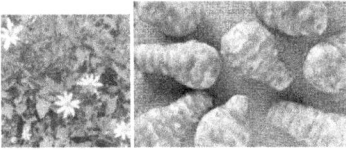

23. **Kale** (collards) is a green leafy vegetable that is a member of the cruciferous or cabbage family. Kale is among the most highly nutritious vegetables. <u>Kale nutrients are used by the thyroid gland along with selenium to make thyroid hormone and therefore increase one's metabolic rate.</u>

    It is an excellent source of carotenes, vitamins A, C, B1, B2, B6 and E. It is also a good source of minerals, manganese, copper, iron and calcium as well as a good source of dietary fiber. *Nutritional and Health info*: See collards and cabbage.

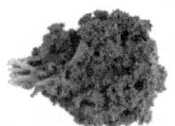

24. **Leeks** (Allium ampeloprasum porrum) belongs to the Amaryllidaceae family, and the subfamily Allioideae. It is related to onions and garlic. *Nutritional and Health info*: All three of these vegetables can <u>lower cholesterol</u> levels, improve the <u>immune system</u>, <u>fight infections</u> and <u>fight cancer.</u>

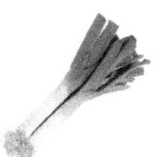

25. **Mustard Greens** (Brassica juncea) is a member of the cabbage or cruciferous family, i.e. broccoli and collards. Mustard greens are a winter plant. They take about 4 to 6 weeks to grow. The Mustard Green plant is a strong plant and does not take a lot of effort to grow.

Nutritional and Health info: of the Mustard Green is worth the effort of growing it. Mustard Greens are one of the most nutritious plants you can eat. In addition to the nutritious greens, this plant also produces the acrid-tasting brown seeds that are used to make Dijon mustard.

Interesting to note is that the Mustard Green seed is mentioned in the Bible and refers to faith being tiny like the mustard seed. Mustard Greens were cultivated in vineyards by the monks who used the very spicy mustard greens and seeds with food for seasoning and nutrition.

The greens contain numerous minerals that seem to render a bitter taste. However, these greens can be helpful in treating asthma and other respiratory problems. The magnesium in mustard greens helps to smooth the walls of the bronchial tubes. Mustard greens also contain several antioxidants, both vitamins A, C, and E and phytonutrients. They are also an excellent source of dietary fiber and protein. Mustard Greens are considered medicinal.

They are believed to fight some cancer cells especially in the colon and stomach. The Mustard Green seed are also known to reduce High Blood Pressure.

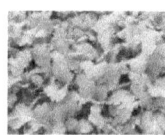

26. **Onions** (Allium cepa), like garlic, are members of the lily family (Amaryllidaceae). <u>Onions as well as garlic are known as a medicinal vegetable.</u>

    Nutritional and Health info: Onions not only block the production of cancer cells they also are known to lower cholesterol, thin the blood and prevent blood clots fight chronic bronchitis, other infections, hay fever and asthma. They are low in calories but relatively moderate in carbohydrates. Onions contain as many as 150 phytonutrients. The flavonoid <u>quercetin</u>, an antioxidant type of phytonutrient that is found in onions, helps eliminate free radicals in the body, thus reducing the risk of cancer, inhibiting low-density lipoprotein (LDL) oxidation, protecting vitamin E, and helping to circumvent the harmful effects of heavy metal ions.

    Other sources of quercetin are tea and apples, but research shows that absorption of quercetin from onions is twice that from tea and more than three times that from apples. Onions are very good for your health. However, they do contaminate your breath, and cause abdominal gas and could be bad for your social life. That could lead to depression which is not good   for your health.

    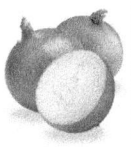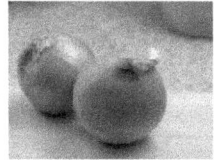

27. **Parsley** (Petroselium crispum) is a member of the Umbelliferae family, just like carrots, parsnips and celery. They share many nutritional and health benefits.

Nutritional and Health info: Parsley contains many nutrients. For instance, they contain calcium, potassium, magnesium, iron, vitamin C, B9 (folic acid), vitamin K, and the phytonutrient beta carotene.

Parsley promotes healthy digestion. Note: Digesting your food efficiently is so essential for good health. This is because digestion of food enables your body to retain and make use of the nutrients from your food. Eating just one sprig of parsley after your meal may keep your digestive system working well and also keep your breathe smelling good and clean. Sprinkling chopped fresh parsley over your food seems to have the same benefits. Eating parsley may also help prevent indigestion and gas. Parsley roots can reduce high blood pressure and reduces chronic inflammation in your body.

Eating parsley can help prevent inflammation throughout the whole body, as well as treat inflammation that has already occurred. Parsley has powerful anti-inflammatory nutrients that may help reverse these dangerous conditions. Remember: Chronic inflammation can lead to many dangerous health conditions. Some of these medical conditions are obesity, diabetes, heart and liver problems, eye and kidney disease, neurological disease, arthritis and even some cancers.

Eating parsley may also help treat allergies by combating the effects of histamine in your body. Parsley may also relieve PMS symptoms and cramping. Parsley is known to have several good detoxify nutrients. Without detoxifying nutrients, a buildup of toxins in your body can lead to illness and disease, and eating parsley may help get rid of those toxins before they pose a health problem.

Parsley contains large amounts of chlorophyll, the agent that results in the dark green color, which acts as a diuretic as well as rids your body of toxins. The human body often contains many foreign chemicals or substances that can lead to many age-related metabolic diseases and some cancers.

Eating parsley may help your body get rid of these toxins more effectively. Just by including parsley at one or two meals a day, you can easily increase your intake of several nutrients. Even a 1-tbsp. sprinkle of parsley can have a good nutritional benefit.

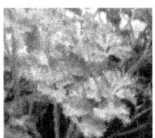

28. **Parsnips** (Pastinaca sativa) like parsley, carrots, and celery, is a member of the Umbelliferae family. They therefore share many health benefits.

   Nutritional and Health info: The parsnip is a root vegetable, and is rich in vitamins and minerals. Sweet and slightly nutty in flavor, pale parsnips are loaded with potassium (like potatoes) and vitamin A (like carrots).

   They also contain folic acid, B vitamins, manganese, copper, magnesium, and fiber, which can help lower your cholesterol and regulate blood sugar. That makes parsnips a healthy addition to your diet, especially at a time of year when your personal nutritional guidelines may be a bit "relaxed," shall we say.

There are about 110 One cup of parsnips contain 110 calories. When peeled they turn dark like potatoes so plan to use them quickly.

Parsnips are usually served boiled or roasted. They can be boiled and mashed like potatoes. You can combine them with carrots, sauté them or add any sweet glaze or roast them together with other winter vegetables.

They can be seasoned with salt, pepper and real butter, olive or coconut oil. They can be used in soups, chowders and stews. Parsnips basically contain the same medicinal properties as carrots and celery.

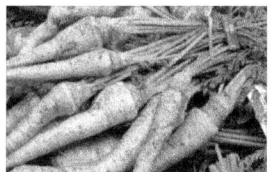

29. **Potatoes** (Solanum tuberosum) is a member of the Solanaceae or nightshade family, whose other members include tomatoes, egg plants and bell peppers. should be included in any balanced diet. Potatoes are a good source of complex, good, carbohydrates and they also provide many other nutrients.

Nutritional and Health info: The carbohydrates in potatoes provide the body with calories that can be used by all cells for energy. Because the body can quickly and effectively break down carbohydrates, which are made up of sugar molecules, they serve as the quick source of energy.

The human body requires many minerals in order to function. Potatoes are a good source of the mineral, Potassium, which is one essential mineral, which is vital for normal heart function, muscle contraction. Potassium also helps to regulate fluid levels and blood pressure.

In addition to potassium, potatoes contain many vitamin C. The body uses vitamin C to support a healthy immune system, protect cells from damage caused by free radicals and produce necessary substances such as collagen -- a group of proteins used to build tendons, ligaments and bones. Potatoes also contain five of the eight B vitamins, including thiamine, niacin, riboflavin, folate and B-6. Potatoes also contain fiber.

Fiber describes the portion of any plant that cannot be broken down during digestion. A high fiber diet promotes a healthy digestive system and reduces blood cholesterol levels, which reduces the risk for heart disease. When consumed with the skin intact, potatoes serve as a good source of fiber.

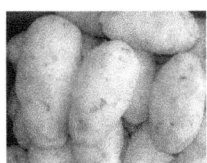

30. **Pumpkins.** A pumpkin is a gourd-like squash of the genus Cucurbita and the family Cucurbitaceae, which also includes gourds and winter squash. They have the same basic *nutritional and health benefits*.

Pumpkins are used in soups, breads, pies and curry sauce ingredients. All pumpkin types provide a variety of nutrients in the diet that supports their use for regular meal planning in addition to special occasion meals.

A 1-cup serving of pumpkin provides 49 calories and 2.7 g of fiber. Including this low-calorie foods in the diet helps you avoid consuming excess calories that contribute to weight gain. Fiber is a nutrient that controls the appetite because it fills you up and controls blood sugar and cholesterol absorption.

Potassium, Vitamin A, lutein, (eye health) Potassium is an important mineral contained in pumpkins and is particularly good for cardiovascular health. It controls the heartbeat contraction. (*Low blood levels of potassium can cause heart arrhythmias*). It also regulates the level of fluid in the bloodstream.

A low level of potassium may cause high blood pressure. Pumpkin improves the heart function and prevents serious cardiovascular disorders. Consuming foods that provide an adequate level of vitamin A helps prevent macular degeneration, a serious eye disease and the leading cause of blindness in the United States.

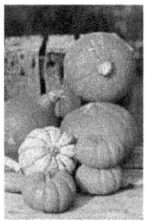

31. **Radishes** (Raphanus sativus) is a root vegetable whose white flesh resembles that of turnips. Like other members

of the cruciferous family, radishes contain a variety of
sulfur-based nutrients that increase the flow of bile.

Radish is a versatile, quick-growing vegetable that can be
grown in a variety of climates. Radishes come in numerous
varieties that can be grown at different times of the year, so
you can enjoy some type of this vegetable at any time.
Having radishes on hand can be beneficial, as this type of
vegetable offers numerous health benefits.

Nutritional and Health info: Also, radishes can be good for
you because they are low in calories. A 100g serving of
radishes contains just 16 calories, which makes this
vegetable ideal for dieting. Radishes are low in fat.
Radishes do not contain any saturated fat or trans fat,
which are types of fat that can increase your risk of
cardiovascular disease.

A diet full of foods low in, saturated fat and devoid of trans
fat can promote heart health. Although radishes are
relatively low in carbohydrates they are rich in fiber, as
nearly half of the carbohydrates in radishes come from
fiber.

Dietary fiber is a nutrient that promotes numerous health
benefits, including stable blood sugar levels, healthy
cholesterol levels and regular bowel movements. Radishes
are rich in potassium, a nutrient that is required for optimal
health because it facilitates contraction of your muscles.
Potassium may also aid in reducing blood pressure and
promoting bone health.

Radishes are healthy because they are rich in calcium, a
nutrient that promotes strong teeth and bones. Calcium, to
the surprise of many, is used by the body to increase

testosterone levels. Radishes are rich in vitamin C, a nutrient that promotes a variety of health benefits. Vitamin C helps heal wounds, produce scar tissue and protects your body from free radical damage.

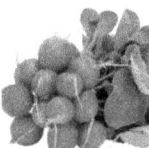

32. **Rutabaga** (Swedish turnip), (Brassica napobrassica) is a root vegetable that originated as a cross between the cabbage and the turnip. The roots are prepared for food in a variety of ways, and its leaves can also be eaten as a leaf vegetable.

Nutritional and Health info: **Rutabaga** is low in sodium, and very low in saturated fat. It is also a good source of dietary fiber, Vitamin A, B1 (Thiamin), B2 (Riboflavin), B3 (Niacin), B5 (Pantothenic acid, B6 (pyridoxine), B9 (folate), C, D, E, and K Mineral such as: Boron, Calcium, Iron, Magnesium and Phosphorus, Potassium, Copper, Zinc, Selenium, Sodium, and Manganese and even fluoride. Rutabaga contains significant amounts of Protein and phytonutrients such as Alpha Tocopherol, Choline, Betaine (like beets).

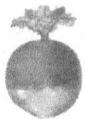

33. **Shallots** (onions) Shallots are considered members of the onion family, but are smaller than onions and look more like garlic. Inside, they do not have concentric structures like onions, but are sectioned into cloves like garlic. The white

flesh can have either red or purple streaks similar to a red or purple onion.

Shallots are strong, rich-tasting and reminiscent of both onions and garlic. Some shallots have coppery brown skin, while others are pinkish or a grayish-brown. Shallots are related to onions, but they have a sweeter, milder flavor. Like garlic and onions, shallots have dry, papery skins. Shallots are native to Israel and regions in the Mediterranean. These flavorful vegetables provide good sources of several important nutrients.

Nutritional and Health info: A ½-cup serving of chopped shallots contains 60 calories and no fat or cholesterol. They do contain Sodium, Carbohydrates, including 3 g of sugars. Shallots are a good source of vitamin A and C. Vitamin C promotes better absorption of iron, and plays an essential role in tooth and gum health, tissue growth and repair and wound healing.

Vitamin A plays an important role in eye and skin health and in the protection against infections. Onions are a good source of iron, a mineral required for the production of hemoglobin. Hemoglobin, a protein found in red blood cells, delivers oxygen to the body's cells, tissues and organs. They also contain calcium. Shallots contain several antioxidant phytochemicals, including phenolics and flavonoids. These phytochemicals have antioxidant and anti-proliferative activities that may protect against cancer. Shallots have a higher phenolic content than many onions, making them particularly effective against liver cancer cells.

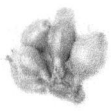

34. **Spinach** (Spinaccia oleracea): Spinach is an edible flowing plant that belongs to the Amaranthaceae, formerly the Chenopodiaceae family. The dark jade-green leaves are higher in nutrient content than virtually any other vegetable food.

    This delicate vegetable is very low in calories and makes a nutritious and makes a colorful addition to any salads. Baby spinach is more tender than regular spinach because it has a higher water content.

    Nutritional and Health info: 2 cups or 6 oz. of raw baby spinach provides 20 calories. It also provides protein, complex carbohydrates and fiber but no fat.. Baby spinach is rich in many micronutrients, as well as vitamins K, A, C and folate: and the minerals iron, calcium, magnesium and potassium.

    Raw spinach needs to be consumed with a few days of picking as many of the vitamins are destroyed. Spinach is rich in vitamin K which is essential for normal blood clotting: it also is important for maintaining bone health.

    Vitamin A is needed for healthy eyesight, proper growth and development and, along with vitamin C, helps supports immune system function.

     Folate is beneficial for both cardiovascular and neurological (brain) health. Spinach is rich in calcium - but it is poorly absorbed by the body because it contains naturally occurring substances known as oxalates.

    Oxalates bind calcium and prevent most of it from being absorbed by the body. Oxalates can also cause kidney stones.

Although spinach is not the best way to meet your calcium requirements, it is still an excellent source of non-heme iron, magnesium and potassium. Iron is essential for oxygen transport throughout the bloodstream and a healthy immune system.

Magnesium, along with vitamin K, is important for maintaining strong, healthy bones, aids in relaxation of muscle and, along with potassium, they all work together to help regulate blood pressure.

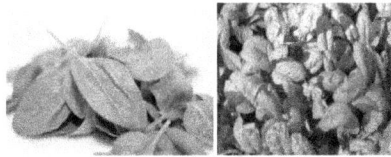

35. **Squash** (summer squash). Yellow summer squash belongs to the Cucurbita pepo family. It is also known as straightneck squash to distinguish it from its close relative, the yellow crookneck squash.

    Yellow squash, also called yellow zucchini or summer squash, is a hot weather vegetable picked in its immature stage to ensure a thin, edible skin and sweet, soft watery flesh. It can be eaten raw, as well as stir-fried, baked, grilled or sautéed, and you can substitute it for any green summer squash since the taste is similar.

    Nutritional and Health Info: One cup of raw, sliced yellow squash contains 18 calories. This low-calorie vegetable is an ideal side dish if you wish to lose weight. Yellow squash essentially has no fat.

Note: eating a low-fat diet may serve as a low-cost preventive measure to ward off breast cancer, according to researchers.

Yellow squash is a good source of healthy complex carbohydrates and fiber. Fiber can play a critical role in helping you lose weight. High-fiber foods satisfy hunger better than low-fiber foods by providing more bulk that stays in your stomach longer. Fiber also helps regulate bowel movements and decreases your chances of developing diverticulitis, a condition that affects your colon.

Everyone should include 25 to 30 g of fiber in their diet every day. Also yellow squash serves as a good source of vitamin C, Ascorbic acid, another name for vitamin C, is an antioxidant that blocks cellular damage from free radicals, helping to slow aging and possibly decreasing your risk of heart disease, arthritis and cancer.

Yellow squash is also a good source of folate, also called folic acid, which is vitamin B9. Not getting enough folate in your diet can result in anemia. However, this vitamin is best known for its role in preventing neurological diseases and preventing birth defects.

Including yellow squash in your meal plan gives a boost in beta carotene. A Beta carotenes are phytonutrients found in the pigments of richly colored fruits and vegetables and some grains.

Yellow squash also provides of manganese, an essential trace mineral required to manufacture sex hormones (i.e., testosterone and estrogen) as well as bones and connective tissues. Also, your body wouldn't have the capability to clot blood without manganese. Manganese along with folate is also used by the body to maintain the normal function of your brain and nerves.

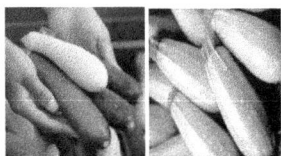

36. **Squash** (winter) acorn, butternut, hubbard, and pumpkin squash.

Nutritional and Health info: This food is very low in Saturated Fat, Cholesterol and Sodium. It is also a good source of Vitamin E (Alpha Tocopherol), Thiamin, Niacin, Vitamin B6, Folate, Calcium and Magnesium, and a very good source of Vitamin A, Vitamin C, Potassium and Manganese.

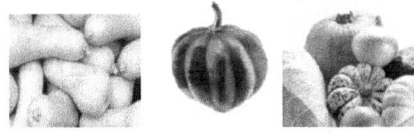

37. **Sweet potatoes** (Ipomoea batatas) is not a member of the potato (Solanaceae) family but rater of the Convolvulaceae, or morning glory family. Although it is sometimes called a yam in North America, the sweet potato is not in the yam family, nor is it closely related to the common potato.

In the U.S., the darker, sweeter, sweet potato is actually a yam. The sweet potato plant is a herbaceous perennial vine, bearing alternate heart-shaped or palmately lobed leaves that are edible. The edible tuberous root is long and tapered, with a smooth skin whose color ranges between yellow, orange, red, brown, purple, and beige. Its flesh ranges from beige through white, red, pink, violet, yellow, orange, and purple. Sweet potato varieties with white or pale yellow flesh are less sweet and moist than those with red, pink or orange flesh.

The plant does not tolerate frost. It grows best at an average temperature of 24 °C, abundant sunshine and warm nights. The crop is sensitive to drought at the tuber initiation stage 50–60 days after planting, and it is not tolerant to water-logging, as it may cause tuber rots and reduce growth of storage roots if aeration is poor. Depending on the cultivar and conditions, tuberous roots mature in two to nine months.

With care, early-maturing cultivars can be grown as an annual summer crop in temperate areas, such as the northern United States. Sweet potatoes are mostly propagated by stem or root cuttings or by adventitious roots called "slips" that grow out from the tuberous roots during storage.

True seeds are used for breeding only. They grow well in many farming conditions and have few natural enemies: pesticides are rarely needed. Sweet potatoes are grown on a variety of soils, but well-drained, light- and medium-textured soils with a pH range of 4.5-7.0 are more favorable for the plant.

They can be grown in poor soils with little fertilizer. However, sweet potatoes are very sensitive to aluminum toxicity and will die about six weeks after planting if lime is not applied at planting in this type of soil.

Because they are sown by vine cuttings rather than seeds, sweet potatoes are relatively easy to plant. Because the rapidly growing vines shade out weeds, little weeding is needed. In the tropics, the crop can be maintained in the ground and harvested as needed for market or home consumption. In temperate regions, sweet potatoes are most often grown on larger farms and are harvested before first frosts.

In the Southeastern United States, sweet potatoes are traditionally cured to improve storage, flavor, and nutrition, and to allow wounds on the periderm of the harvested root to heal. Proper curing requires drying the freshly dug roots on the ground for two to three hours, then storage at 85–90 °F) with 90 to 95% relative humidity from five to fourteen days. Cured sweet potatoes can keep for thirteen months when stored at 55–59 °F. Colder temperatures injure the root .

Nutritional and Health info: Sweet potatoes are an excellent source of carotenes as well as a good source of vitamins A, C and B2, B3, B5, B6 and dietary fiber. It is also a good source of manganese, and copper. Sweet potatoes also contain a storage protein called Dioscorin. Dioscorin is a protein that can help your body to achieve increased kidney blood flow thereby reducing blood pressure.

In addition, sweet potatoes are good sources of complex carbohydrates and fiber which deliver the sugar and cholesterol in the intestines gradually into the blood stream. This slows the rate at which their sugars and cholesterol are released and absorbed into the bloodstream.

Because they're rich in fiber, sweet potatoes fill you up without filling out your hips and waistline. Sweet potatoes are also a good source of manganese, a trace mineral that helps with carbohydrate metabolism and is a cofactor in a number of enzymes important in energy production and antioxidant defenses and producing hormones.

Sweet potatoes are considered an 'anti-diabetic' food because the help stabilize blood sugar levels and improve the response to the insulin hormone.

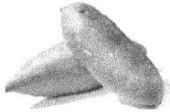

38. **Swiss Chard** (Beta vulgaris cicla) is a member of the same family as beets and spinach (Chenopodiaceae). See Chard above.

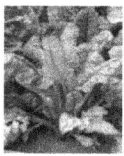

39. **Tomatoes** are a member of the Solanaceae or nightshade family along with bell peppers, eggplant, and potatoes.

Nutritional and Health info: the tomato is a low-calorie food packed with nutrition, especially when fully ripe. They are an excellent source of phyto-nutrients, especially the beta carotene, lycopene. Tomatoes are also an excellent source of Vitamins B3, B5, B6, B7, B9, and vitamin C and K. It is also a good source of dietary fiber.

Lycopene is a red carotene phyto-nutrient that has been shown to protect against breast cancer, colon, lung, shin, and prostate cancers. Also it has been shown to lower the risk of heart disease, cataracts, and macular degeneration. Lycopene helps prevent these diseases and others by neutralizing harmful oxygen free radicals before they can do damage to cellular structures.

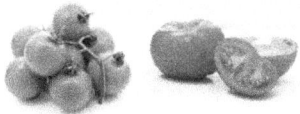

40. **Turnips** and **Turnip Greens** (Brassica rapa rapifeera) are members of the cruciferous vegetable family. Both the root and the greens of turnips are edible. Turnip greens are smaller and tenderer than their cousin, collards, and they have a slightly bitter flavor.

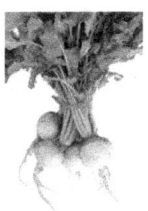

41. **Yam**. The true yam is a member of the Dioscoreaceae family and are different for the sweet potatoes labeled "yams".

Nutrition and Health info: Yams are a good source of both potassium and vitamin B6, two nutrients that your body needs every day. Vitamin B6 helps your body break down a substance called homocysteine, which can cause damage to blood vessel walls and is a known risk factor for heart disease.

High intakes of vitamin B6 have been shown to reduce the risk of heart disease. Potassium is a mineral that helps to control blood pressure. Yams also contain a storage protein called Dioscorin. Preliminary research suggests that Dioscorin can help your body to achieve increased kidney blood flow thereby reducing blood pressure.

In addition, Yams' complex carbohydrates and fiber deliver the goods gradually, slowing the rate at which their sugars are released and absorbed into the bloodstream. Because they're rich in fiber, yams fill you up without filling out your hips and waistline.

Yams are also a good source of manganese, a trace mineral that helps with carbohydrate metabolism and is a cofactor in a number of enzymes important in energy production and antioxidant defenses.

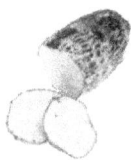

CHAPTER 5   NUTS, SEEDS AND VEGETABLE OILS

Nuts and Seeds contain macro- and micro-nutrients. The macro-nutrients are the caloric nutrients: i.e., fats, proteins, and carbohydrates. The micro-nutrients are the minerals, vitamins, and phytonutrients. The micronutrients that are organic are called phytonutrients (phyto-chemicals) or medicinal nutrients (medicinal chemicals).

Nuts are dry fruits or seeds with a hard shell and a firm inner kernel or shell enclosed seeds. Nuts and seeds are an excellent source for nutritional chemicals, being especially good sources of essential fatty acids, vitamin E, protein, and minerals.

Because of their high oil content, nuts and seeds are often used as sources of oils for use in culinary, medicinal, and cosmetic preparation. <u>The coconut is the most widely grown and utilized nut crop, followed by the peanut</u>. One of the main reasons is that coconuts and peanuts provide oils that are among the leading ingredients of cooking oils.

For the cook as well as the health expert, oils are a healthy and necessary ingredient. They add fat for browning and for consistency, and many oils add flavor and nutritional chemicals to our food. Oils derived from nuts and seeds also contribute to a well-balanced diet.

Fats such as monounsaturated, polyunsaturated, and saturated fats are all present in nut and seed oils. These technical terms refer to the molecular structure of the oil, more specifically, to the number of hydrogen atoms present. Saturated fats, the least healthy, contain the maximum possible number of hydrogen atoms. The healthier polyunsaturated and monounsaturated fats have less than their maximum of hydrogen atoms, so they combine more easily with other substances within the body to form structures.

Olive oil is high in monounsaturated fats, while palm and coconut oils have the highest levels of saturated fats. Although there are general-purpose oils these can generally be divided into cooking oils-those that are fairly neutral in flavor and withstand heat well and seasoning oils, which are best used to flavor uncooked dishes such as salads. Popular low cost cooking oils include soy and corn oils. Walnut and hazelnut oils can be heated, but are most successful as seasoning oils because these oils are expensive.

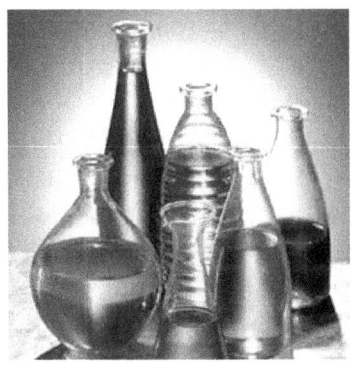

A guide to the usefulness of cooking oils.

Cooking oil is plant, animal, or synthetic fat used in frying, baking, and other types of cooking. It is also used in food preparation and flavoring that doesn't involve heat, such as salad dressings and bread dips, and in this sense might be more accurately termed edible oil.

Cooking oil is typically a liquid, although some oils that contain saturated fat, such as coconut oil, palm oil and palm kernel oil, are solid at room temperature.

 Types of cooking oil include: olive oil, palm oil, soybean oil, canola oil (rapeseed oil), pumpkin seed oil, corn oil, sunflower oil, safflower oil, peanut oil, grape seed oil, sesame oil, rice bran oil and other vegetable oils. Oil can be flavored with aromatic foodstuffs such as nuts, herbs, chilies or garlic.

Types of edible oils

1.   Almond Oil is a pale oil made from sweet almonds. It is used in baking and confectionery. It is good for coating cake pans or cookie sheets when preparing delicate baked goods.

2.   Avocado Oil is extracted from the pits of avocados, and sometimes from blemished fruit. This oil is colorless with a faint aniseed flavor. It is used mainly in North America.

3.   Canola Oil is also known as rapeseed oil. This oil is a neutral-flavored oil that is suitable for frying, cooking, or baking. It has a high smoke point and is low in saturated fats.

4.   Coconut Oil is extracted from the dried kernel of the coconut. Coconut oil is often used in commercial food preparations and in certain Indian dishes. It is high in saturated fats.

5.   Corn Oil is one of the most economical and widely used all-purpose oils. This oil has a deep yellow in color and is heavy in texture. Corn oil is high in polyunsaturated fats and has a high smoke point, so it is both healthy and ideal for both cooking and salads.

6.   Cottonseed Oil is derived from the cotton plant. This oil is used in the hydrogenation process for the production of margarine and shortening.

7.   Grapeseed Oil is a pale, delicate oil extracted from grape seeds. This oil can withstand a wide range of temperatures. When refrigerated, it will not cloud, making it ideal for the oil constituent of mayonnaise. Also, it has a very high smoke point so it is excellent for frying and cooking in general. It is also high in polyunsaturated fats.

8. Hazelnut Oil is a delicious, richly flavored oil that is extracted from the hazelnut. It is produced mainly in France and is very expensive. It should be used with the finest vinegars for salad dressings, or as a marinade for fish or poultry. Its delicate flavor is lost when heated, but it can be whisked into a sauce at the last minute or used in some baked goods in combination with hazelnuts.

9. Palm Oil is also known as palm nut oil. This oil is extracted from the pulp of the fruit of oil palms. It is orange-gold in color and has a pleasant nutty flavor. It is considered a general-purpose oil because it has a light taste and color as well as it is good for frying and making salad dressings. It does, however, turn rancid very rapidly and should be stored in the refrigerator.

10. Peanut Oil is a very fine, almost tasteless oil that is good for general use in salads, cooking, and frying. The cold-pressed variety has a mild peanut flavor that is good with fruit-flavored vinegars for salad dressings. Also, peanut oil is a healthy oil because it is moderately high in mono-unsaturates and low in saturates.

11. Pine Seed Oil has a distinctive pine seed flavor. This oil is produced on a small scale primarily in France. It is very expensive but is known to have a great flavor. It is best used in salads.

12. Pumpkin Seed Oil is a dark brown oil with a pleasant flavor of toasted pumpkin seeds. It is produced in Austria. It is especially good as a seasoning for steamed vegetables or fish.

13. Safflower Oil has a bright yellow color and is ideal for all culinary use even though it has a rather strong flavor. This

cooking oil is the highest in polyunsaturated fats, lowest in saturated fats, and is a good source of vitamin E.

14.   Sesame Oil has many types. European, or cold-pressed sesame oil, is a good cooking oil because it has a high smoke point and a nutty flavor. Asian sesame oil is made from toasted sesame seeds, giving it a darker color and more pronounced taste. Middle Eastern sesame oils are lighter in flavor than Asian ones, with a deep golden color. All are aromatic and capable of being heated to high temperatures because of their relatively high smoke point.

15.   Soy Oil is a major component of blended oils that are high-quality, neutral-flavored oils. They are low in saturated fats. They have a high smoke point so can be used for frying, cooking or on salads.

16.   Sunflower Oil is one of the best all-purpose oils. It is high in polyunsaturates, tasteless, pale, light in texture, and inexpensive. It can be used for frying, cooking, salad dressings, and mixing with other more strongly flavored oils.

17. Vegetable Oil is an oil obtained from blending a number of oils in various proportions, and types and quantities are not necessarily given on the label. It may contain coconut or palm oils, which are high in saturated fats. Vegetable oil has little aroma or flavor, making it popular as an all-purpose culinary oil.

18. Walnut Oil has a beautiful topaz-color with a rich, nutty flavor. It is produced from the best grade of walnuts. Walnut oil is expensive. Walnut oil does not keep long, either opened or unopened which is one of the reasons it is so expensive. Also, it must be kept in cool places at all times: but not in the refrigerator. It does make a delicious salad dressing, and adds

the walnut flavor to cakes and cookies, especially those that contain walnuts. .

Nut and Seed Oils are especially popular for adding flavor to foods.

Nut and seed oils are generally used as a flavoring for cold food, or added to hot dishes at the last minute. Pumpkin seed, walnut and hazelnut oils, Asian sesame oil, cold-pressed peanut and pine seed oils all make superb salad dressings, vegetable seasonings, and marinades. They should always be used sparingly and in combination with a neutral oil, such as sun-flower, because their flavor is sometimes overpowering. They can also be used much the same as a pat of butter, to flavor cooked foods. Walnut oil can be tossed over steamed or boiled green beans just before serving.

Oils with a distinct taste should be chosen in order to enhance particular dishes. Often they are too overpowering to be used simply for general-purpose cooking. Such oils, particularly if they are not blended, tend also to be expensive so they are best used where only a small amount is needed.

Examples of nuts and seeds and their nutritional value as food nutrients:

1. **Almonds** are high in vitamin E, a powerful anti-oxidant micronutrient. The addition of almonds to your daily diet can help lower levels of LDL cholesterol, also known as "bad" cholesterol: they can increase your daily intake of numerous important nutrients: and they can help you maintain or achieve a healthy weight. Almonds are known as a super-food because of their nutritional content. Almonds contain high levels of monounsaturated fat, which helps lower LDL cholesterol levels and thus lowers the risk of heart disease. Most of the carbohydrates in

almonds are in the form of fiber (a good thing). Almonds are also a good source of complete protein. The amount of protein in a serving of almonds is greater than an egg. In addition, almonds are a cholesterol-free food, which isn't the case with many complete protein sources, such as eggs and meat.

Almonds are a good source of vitamins. These include the B vitamins: vitamin B1 (thiamin), B2 (riboflavin), B3 (niacin), B7 (biotin) as well as vitamin E. Vitamin E is an important antioxidant that protects cells in the body from free radicals, especially those in the skin, heart and red blood cells. In addition, almonds contain a variety of essential minerals such as calcium, copper, iron, magnesium, manganese, phosphorous, potassium and zinc.

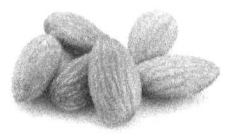

Almonds are a good source of nutrients: especially for vegetarians who have a hard time reaching their daily requirements for calcium and iron as well as for their complete protein.

2. **Brazil nuts:** high in the mineral selenium: an important mineral for thyroid function and wound healing. They are high in good omega 3 and omega 6 fatty acids. Although they pack in fat, Brazil nuts have many healthy minerals such as: calcium, iron, magnesium, copper, manganese and a large amount of selenium. Selenium is a trace mineral that is essential for many enzymes to function properly, especially in the respiratory system, skin (integumentary system) or wound healing and thyroid gland functioning. Brazil nuts are known to benefit those individuals with

Asthma. Brazil nuts are low in sodium. This especially
makes Brazil nuts good for snacking
because naturally low-sodium foods
are almost unheard of among
snacks. Unlike most snacks, Brazil
nuts don't contain empty calories
and are considered a high-protein food.

3. **Cashew nuts**: though cashews are high in fat, it is
unsaturated fat, which is healthier than saturated fat. This
type of fat can help lower blood cholesterol levels and
reduce your risk for developing chronic diseases, such as
heart disease.

Nutritional Facts: Cashews and other nuts are great sources
of protein and make suitable substitutes for meat. In
addition to protein, cashews contain vitamin E and the
minerals phosphorus, zinc, magnesium and selenium, all of
which are nutrients required for good health.

One serving of cashews, equal to 1 oz. or approximately 14
cashews and provides 180 to 200 calories. Cashews are
delicious enjoyed by themselves as a snack, and their sweet,
buttery flavor makes them decadent enough to have as an
appetizer when entertaining guests.

They are especially good added to yogurt or breakfast

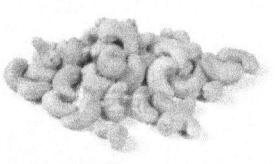

granola, or sprinkled on top of a
salad for lunch or dinner. They can
also be delicious as a stir-fry
ingredient. Always choose plain,
unsalted nuts. Dry-roasted
versions with added salt contain up to 179 mg sodium per
ounce. Cashews come from trees related to mangoes,

pistachios, and sumac. Cashew nuts have the following nutrients: folate, beta-carotene, vitamin K, phosphorus, copper, selenium, zinc and potassium. Cashews, like other nuts, are both calorie and nutrient dense and can play a role in a healthy diet.

4. **Chestnuts** are most frequently associated with Christmas, as a seasonal treat. Chestnuts are lower in fat and protein than other types of nuts, but they are higher in fiber, making them a nutritious choice for a morning or afternoon snack. One half cup of roasted chestnuts have 175 calories, 3.6 g of dietary fiber and 7.5 g of sugars which is a good fiber/sugar ratio.

    Chestnuts are a complete source of the nine amino acids your body needs but must get from food, called essential amino acids. Chestnuts are also high in nonessential amino acids your body can produce, including aspartic acid and glutamic acid.

    Chestnuts are fairly low in fat compared to other nuts. They contain only 5-6 calories of saturated fats, with no trans fats or cholesterol. In addition, they 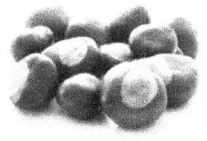 contain 18 calories of unsaturated fats, which are considered healthy, omega 3 and omega 6 fatty acids that can help lower your cholesterol. Chestnuts are also high in vitamins and minerals, especially potassium and chestnuts are high in antioxidants such as: vitamin C, vitamin A and the phytonutrient, leucine. Finally, chestnuts are rich in the vitamin K and the B family, especially (B9) folate.

5. **Coconuts:** One cup of raw coconut contains about 300 calories, 7g of dietary fiber and 21g of carbohydrates. The total fat content is about 30g. The fat is a type of saturated fat and is known as a <u>medium chain fatty acids</u> (MCFA). <u>MCFA are rare</u> and basically found only in coconut oil. <u>This type of fat is more beneficial to good health than the long chain fatty acids</u>.

Also, MCFA are digested by the body in a different way than the common long chain fatty acids (LCFA) found in most other foods. Because they are quickly digested, <u>MCFA produce energy instead of body fat. Also MCFA are less likely to produce arterial plaque like other saturated fats</u>.

Most of the medium-chain fatty acids (oils) in coconuts are omega 3 and omega 6 fatty acids in the form of lauric acid and cyprylic acid. Lauric acid is the same kind of fat found in 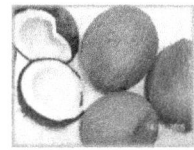 human breast milk and lauric acid is known to strengthen the human immune system.

The caprylic acid is a type of fat that has antifungal, antiviral and antibacterial properties. The highest vitamin source of vitamins is folate. Other vitamins in coconut include vitamin C, and vitamin E, thiamine (B1), riboflavin (B2), niacin (3), pantothenic acid (B5) and B6 (pyroxidine). Raw coconut is a rich source of minerals such as: <u>manganese, copper, selenium</u> and <u>iron</u>. Also, raw coconut is low in sodium.

6. **Flaxseeds (Linseeds)**: Flaxseed consists of small, golden-colored seed derived from the flax plant. It is known for its unique <u>nutty taste and a distinct chewy texture</u>.

    Nutritional and Health Info: Flaxseed is known for its high nutritional. Flaxseed is also an abundant source of essential macro and micro-nutrient like: <u>protein</u>, <u>soluble fiber</u>, <u>phytonutrients</u> (i.e., lignans that act as plant estrogens), <u>vitamin B9 (folic acid)</u>, <u>magnesium, potassium, calcium and iron</u> and a type of <u>omega-3 fatty acid called alpha-linolenic acid</u>.

    Flaxseed is known to promote healthy digestive function, to boost cardiovascular performance and to help discourage the growth of cancerous tumors. Flaxseed's high soluble fiber content enables it to act like a laxative and can be used to help relieve uncomfortable constipation.

    The (ALA) alpha-linolenic acid found in flaxseed has the ability to help lower bad cholesterol levels and decrease your risk of heart disease. Flaxseed is sold in packages of whole seeds that you can eat right out of the box or in pre-ground form.

    You can sprinkle flaxseed on top of your oatmeal or mixing it in with yogurt, fruit smoothies and/or protein shakes. You can also add flaxseed to baked products like breads muffins and other pastries. Flaxseeds exhibit very few side effects.

    Due to high fiber content however, flaxseed does have the potential to cause diarrhea. Therefore, you should be especially careful about flaxseed consumption if you suffer from a digestive disorder like frequent diarrhea or Crohn's disease. Also, <u>keep in mind that the high fiber content can interfere with the absorption of many medications and/or nutritional supplements.</u>

7. **Hazelnuts:** are a sweet in taste and incredibly nutritious nut. They are in the same family as the birch tree, the Betulaceae family of trees. Hazelnut oil has a nutty aroma. The oil is used in cooking, and as "base oil" in medicines, in massage therapy, aromatherapy, in pharmaceutical and in the cosmetic industry.

Nutritional and Health Info: Hazelnuts are a very good source of energy and essential nutrients. One cup of hazelnuts contains approximately 650 calories. The nuts are rich in mono-unsaturated fatty acids like oleic as well as essential fatty acid, linoleic acid.

The mono-unsaturated fatty acids (oleic) and linoleic acid are known to lower LDL (the bad cholesterol) and increase HDL (the good cholesterol). Hazelnuts therefore help to prevent coronary artery disease and strokes. These nuts are rich in dietary fiber, vitamins, and minerals and phyto-chemicals. Altogether, they help protect from diseases and cancers. Hazelnuts are exceptionally rich in folate. Folate is an important vitamin that helps prevent megaloblastic anemia and most importantly, neural tube defects in the newborn as well as <u>prevents or slows down memory loss associated with dementia in adults.</u>

The folate in hazelnuts is even considered to be effective in slowing down Alzheimer's disease and Parkinson's disease. Hazel nuts are an excellent source of vitamin E, which is a powerful lipid soluble antioxidant, required for maintaining the integrity of cell membranes.

Anti-oxidants protect the body from harmful oxygen-free radicals by neutralizing and therefore rendering them "neutral". The nuts are packed with many important B-vitamins such as thiamine (B1), riboflavin (B2), niacin (B3), pantothenic acid (B5), pyridoxine (B-6), and folates (B9).

They are rich source of minerals like manganese, potassium, calcium, copper, magnesium, iron, zinc, and selenium. Note: copper, zinc, iron and manganese are essential co-factors for the superoxide dismutase enzyme, an enzyme necessary for longevity and the prevention of some cancers and neurological diseases. Iron helps prevent microcytic-anemia. Folic acid (B9) prevents macrocytic anemia.

8. **Macadamia nuts**: These nuts are very low in cholesterol and sodium. They also are a good source of vitamin B1 (Thiamine), and Manganese. Macadamia nuts have a pleasant buttery taste and crisp, light texture and these nuts are loaded with healthy nutrients.

    Nutritional and Health info: One ounce of Macadamia Nuts contains 200 calories. They have both monounsaturated fat and saturated fat, 17g to 3g for a total of 20 grams of fat per one once serving. They contain 4 g of carbohydrates, 2 g of fiber and 1 gram of sugar and 1 gram of protein.

    The Macadamia nut contains minerals such as Manganese, Magnesium, Copper, Phosphorus, Iron, Zinc, Potassium and Vitamin B1 (thiamine), B3 (Niacin), and B6 (pyrodxidine. Although these nuts are high in fat, it's the healthy monounsaturated fats that dominate.

They are known to have higher levels of mono-unsaturated fats than any natural, commercially available food source. This type of fat can lower the risk of heart disease by enhancing good cholesterol (HDL), while helping to suppress and lower the bad cholesterol (LDL).

Macadamia nuts are a good source of protein. They contain all of the essential amino acids as well as some non-essential amino acids. Protein is important for muscle growth and repair, as well as supports a healthy immune system.

 The carbohydrates in macadamia nuts include sugars, such as fructose, glucose, sucrose and maltose, as well as a quantity of other starchy substances. These carbohydrates are necessary for energy.

The fiber in macadamia nuts helps to give a feeling of fullness and reduces hunger pangs. Fiber is also important for digestion. It helps to maintain the health of your intestines by promoting the right balance of intestinal bacteria and can aid in relieving constipation.

Macadamias contain important antioxidants, such as vitamin E and selenium, as well as many phytonutrients. These essential nutrients are free radical scavengers: they can help to prevent free radical damage in the body. The monounsaturated fats contained in macadamia nuts are thought to metabolize differently from other types of fats.

Many studies show that nut eaters usually weigh less than those that don't eat nuts. Substituting macadamia nuts for other high fat snacks will lead to safe and effective weight loss. Because their shells are hard to crack, they are usually purchased shelled. They are found both in their raw state or roasted state and either salted or unsalted.

It's best to purchase macadamia nuts in airtight containers because the high fat content of macadamia nuts can become rancid and harmful. Unopened containers may be stored in the refrigerator for up to six months, or in the freezer for up to a year.

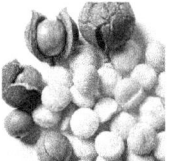

Once the nuts are opened, it's best to keep them in the refrigerator and consume them within two months. Macadamia nuts should be light in color. If they start to darken, that's a sign that they are starting to turn rancid and it's best to through them away.

9. **Olives**: There are many different types of olives and the broad categories are the green olives and the ripe black olives. The nutritional value of olives stems from the fact that they have <u>very little carbohydrate</u> and are a great source of mono-unsaturated fat. This makes it a good for any low-carb diet. Olives are a rich source of several important phytonutrients.

One of these phytonutrients are the <u>polyphenols which are critical for our body's defense against cancer</u>.

Polyphenols have many good nutrient properties. They are the reason for the taste and the smell of the olives. Some of the polyphenols in olives act as anti-oxidants and some act as anti-inflammatory nutrients.

The following is a list of the variety of nutrients that we can get from a small amount of olives. A normal serving of olives is considered to be 10 medium sized green olives.

Olives contains Water, 49 calories, protein, carbohydrate, fat, carbohydrates, sugars, fiber and monounsaturated fatty acids and polyunsaturated fatty acids.

Olives also contain minerals such as Calcium, Copper, Iron, Magnesium, Phosphorus, Potassium, Selenium, Sodium, Zinc. The list of vitamins include: vitamins A, B1 (thiamine), B2 (riboflavin, B3 (Niacin), B-6 (pyridoxine), B9 (folate), vitamin E (alpha tocopherol) and vitamin K.

This list of phyto-nutrients includes: Beta Carotene, Beta Cryptoxanthin, Lutein, Zeaxanthin and Choline. Olive oil, which is extracted by pressing oils from olives, is a good source of many beneficial nutrients.

The oil is not only a good source of antioxidants it also greatly adds to the flavor of dishes. As it contains monounsaturated fat, it does not elevate the level of cholesterol in the body as such olive oil can prevent the adherence of cholesterol to the walls of the artery.

Additionally, monosaturated fats also help in controlling blood sugar. This affects the insulin regulatory system in the body in a positive way. It is best to choose cold-pressed olive oil because heated processing erodes some of the best benefits of this oil.

 Extra virgin olive oil, which refers to the first pressed oil, is considered the healthiest. Extra virgin olive oil has the least amount of acidity. While olive oil is fairly stable and does not become rancid like some other cooking oils, it is still best to not store too much of the oil at home unless it is refrigerated. If you are buying canned olives, they can technically be stored for up to two years if they are unopened. Olives can be dry-cured and stored in a refrigerator.

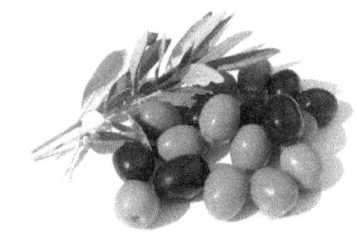

10. **Peanuts** are part of the dried bean and legume family. They are a cholesterol-free, whole food, containing many vitamins and minerals, including vitamin E and potassium.

Nutritional Fact: Peanuts are rich in niacin (vitamin B3) which is known to lowers cholesterol. Peanuts are also a good source of protein. They provide more plant protein than any other nut or legume.

The following is a list of some of the other nutrients found in peanuts: protein, monounsaturated fat, polyunsaturated fat, omega-6 fatty acids and trace amounts of omega-3 fatty acids.

Peanuts not only contain niacin (B3), they also contain folate (B9), and (pyridoxine) (B6), dietary fiber as well as adequate amounts of zinc, copper, iron and magnesium.

Peanut oil is a good cooking oil as it can be heated to high temperatures. ***The smoke point of an oil or fat is the*** *temperature at which it begins to break down to glycerol and free fatty acids, and produce bluish smoke.*

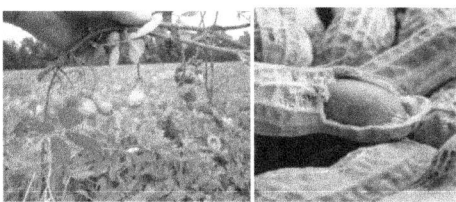

11. **Pecans:** <u>pecans and walnuts</u> provide similar nutritional profiles, as both are calorie-dense nuts that are high in good fats. Despite these similarities, the two have a number of nutritional differences: even the characteristics that are similar.

    For instance, the fat and calorie content vary depending on the nut. Walnuts and pecans can both be healthy choices, but you may find one preferable, depending on your individual tastes and nutritional needs.

    If you're dieting, <u>walnuts</u> would be a slightly better choice than pecans, as walnuts contain 185 calories per 1-oz. serving, while pecans provide 196. If you're active, however, this difference may not be significant as you can burn off the extra 15 calories in 1 oz. of pecans through less than two minutes of jogging.

    As with other types of nuts, pecans and walnuts are both rich in fat. Pecans are higher in fat, with 20 g per 1-oz. serving, compared to 18.5 g in 1 oz. of walnuts. Both pecans and walnuts are low in saturated fat.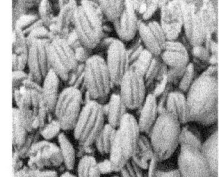

Both pecans and walnuts are rich sources of dietary fiber. Fiber helps you feel full, promotes regular bowel movements and aids in digestion. Pecans and walnuts are both relatively low in protein, but walnuts contain more of this important nutrient. Neither is a rich source of protein.

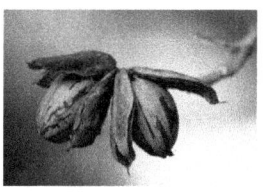 Pecans contain much more zinc than walnuts. Zinc is essential for optimal health, as it facilitates the proper functioning of many enzymes and is a structural component of proteins and cell membranes: it is also believed to aid in the treatment of viral and fungal infections.

Walnuts contain nearly five times the folate that pecans provide. Folate is vitamin B9 and is especially important for pregnant women and nursing 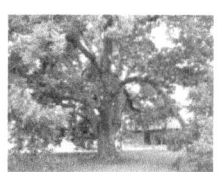 mothers, because it can help prevent anemia and because it encourages proper growth of new cells especially nerve cells. Folate is also important in treating most neurological diseases i.e. senile dementia and memory loss and even slow the progression of Alzheimer's disease.

12. **Pine nuts**: Pine nuts are edible seeds from pine trees, popularly used in pesto sauces, as a food topping, in desserts, and in meat and fish dishes. Pine nuts have 53 calories per one-tablespoon serving and are low in cholesterol, sodium and sugar but high in protein.

    Pine nuts are high in fat: monounsaturated fat: polyunsaturated fat: and saturated fat. Pine nuts contain vitamin B-6 (pyridoxine), vitamin E and vitamin K. Pine nuts are a good source of magnesium, and calcium. Other minerals found in high quantities are of phosphorus and potassium.

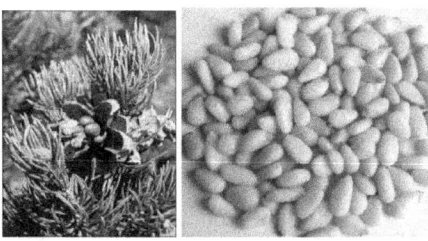

13. **Pistachio nuts:** Pistachios are <u>among the most nutritious of nuts</u> you can choose. They offer more fiber and fewer calories than many other varieties, including almonds, cashews, walnuts and macadamias. Pistachios make a healthy snack because of their healthy fats, fiber and taste. A <u>1 oz.</u> serving of pistachio nuts is considered the normal serving size. It consists of 50 nuts and about 160 calories.

Pistachio nuts also provide unsaturated fats carbohydrates, proteins ad numerous essential vitamins and minerals and phytonutrients. Pistachios as well as almonds provide more protein per serving of any nuts.

The following is a list of some of the essential vitamins, minerals and phytonutrients. Vitamin A, C, E, B-1, B-6, niacin (B-3), folate (B-9) and riboflavin (B-2): Calcium, iron, phosphorus, zinc, manganese, selenium, copper and potassium.

Remember: potassium helps with fluid and mineral balance as well as cardiovascular health benefits. Other benefits are the phytonutrients in Pistachios which are <u>phyto-sterols</u>, compounds found in plants that deter your body from absorbing dietary cholesterol: lutein, an antioxidant that helps with <u>eye</u> and skin health and <u>fights free radicals that promote aging</u>.

One serving (50 nuts) of pistachios is a good source of fiber. Also, pistachios nuts can raise one's metabolic rate. This is important for the breaking down of food in order to release its nutrients and energy (i.e., metabolism). Ounce for ounce, pistachios are much healthier than fries or chips

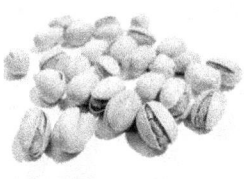 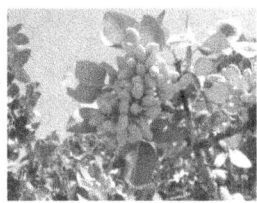

14. **Pumpkin Seeds** (Cucurbita pepo): Pumpkin seeds are also called pepitas. Pumpkin seeds are commonly roasted and salted for a snack or garnish, or used as a crust for fish or chicken. Pumpkin seeds, whether roasted at home or purchased hulled, make a nutritious snack. One fourth cup of roasted pumpkin seeds is considered the normal serving size that contains about 170 calories.

They serve as a good source of protein and fiber. Most of the fat in an ounce of pumpkin seeds is the unsaturated variety. A list of other nutrients found in pumpkin seeds is: <u>magnesium</u>, <u>iron</u>, <u>manganese</u>, <u>copper</u> and <u>zinc</u>.

Pumpkin seeds like sunflower seeds and pistachio nuts are high in phyto-sterols, compounds that are known to help reduce cholesterol levels, enhance immunity and decrease the risk of developing certain cancers.

Pumpkin seeds can be enjoyed year-round. Just scoop them out of a pumpkin, rinse off the membrane, coat with cooking spray or olive oil and bake in a 250 degree F oven for an hour, stirring them every 10 to 15 minutes. Flavor them with chili powder, cumin (mustard) and salt, garlic salt or cinnamon sugar.

They are very good and savory in a salad with avocado, grapefruit and romaine lettuce. Sweetly flavored versions can be mixed into a cream cheese for a spread on bagels or toast, or used as a topping for pudding or ice cream. Add them to granola or popcorn for extra nutrition and texture.

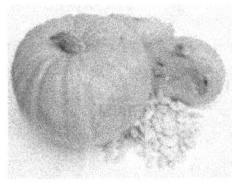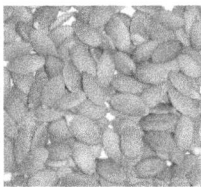

15. **Sesame Seeds** (Sesamum indicum): Sesame seeds have been used for their nutrition, crunch and for their oil since 1600 B.C. Sesame seed oil is known for being "exceptionally resistant to rancidity," a key factor for safety and health.

    Sesame seeds play an important role in many foods. They add texture to Asian dishes, as well as all breads and bagels. While sesame seeds are small, they still have nutritional facts to consider. *Nutritional Info*: One ounce of sesame seeds is high in calcium, iron, and dietary fiber. Also, sesame seeds can be a significant source of protein and fat if used in abundance.

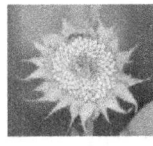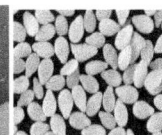

16. **Sunflower Seeds**: There are many options for sunflower seeds--shelled or unshelled, salted or unsalted, plain or flavored. Raw sunflower seeds are the most natural form. These tiny seeds contain an excellent source of nutrients. Sunflower seeds are a calorie-dense food. A one ounce serving (two teaspoons) provide 165 calories. A one ounce serving is considered to be equal to two tablespoons. This serving size contains 22 calories and is a good source of protein.

Seeds are actually classified as fitting into the "Meats and Beans" category of the USDA's Food Guide Pyramid. Because of their protein content, seeds like sunflower seeds are a popular protein source for vegetarian and vegan diets. Sunflower seeds also provide good fats. Most of the fat is unsaturated good fat and is liquid at room temperature. In contrast, saturated fat "bad fat" is most commonly from hydrogenated oils (trans-fats) or animal sources. Saturated fats are solid at room temperature.

Replacing saturated with unsaturated fat can lower your total and low-density (LDL) cholesterol, which lowers your risk for heart disease. Not only are sunflower seeds packed with protein and healthy fat, they provide other essential nutrients.

Sunflower seeds are an excellent source of vitamin E. One of the best known roles of vitamin E is that it acts as an anti-oxidant. Remember: anti-oxidants protect cells from damage by free radicals by neutralizing them and making them non-reactive and neutral.

Vitamin E also works to boost your immune system. Also, vitamin E research shows it has a positive effect on preventing cancer, heart disease, eye disorders and mental function. In addition to vitamin E, sunflower seeds contain a variety of minerals and vitamins. A serving of seeds provides vitamin B6 (pyridoxine) which plays an important role in red cell metabolism, protein metabolism and nervous and immune system functioning.

 Sunflower seeds are also a good source of some important mineral: i.e., iron, which is essential for the development of hemoglobin. Hemoglobin helps carry oxygen in the blood and selenium.

Selenium works with protein to make seleno-proteins, some of which <u>act as antioxidants</u>, while other seleno-proteins <u>regulate thyroid function and assist in strengthening the immune function</u>. Sunflower seeds can be sprinkled on salads or mixed with nuts and dried fruit for a hardy trail mix. They can also be added on top of a vegetable side dish for an added crunch. Remember that it is best to choose the unsalted variety to limit your sodium intake.

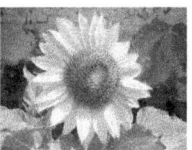 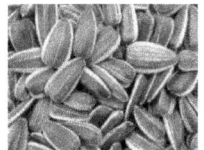

17. **Walnuts:** (Class Magnoliopsida, Order Fagales, Family Juglandaceae, Genus Juglans, Species regia) The two most common major species of walnuts, the English Walnut and the Black Walnut. Walnuts are grown for their edible seeds (the nut).

The Black walnut is considered to have the best flavor, but due to its hard shell and poor hulling characteristics it is not grown commercially for nut production. The commercially produced walnut varieties are nearly all hybrids of the English walnut.

Walnuts secrete chemicals into the soil to prevent competing vegetation from growing. Because of this, flowers or vegetable gardens should not be planted too close to them.

The husks of walnut contains a juice that will readily stain anything it comes into contact with: therefore its juice has been used as a dye for cloth.

The Nutritional and Health Info is very similar to pecans. (see Pecans info above). Walnut seeds are a high density source of nutrients, particularly proteins and essential fatty acids. Walnuts, like other tree nuts, must be processed and stored properly. Poor storage makes walnuts susceptible to insect and fungal-mold infestations. It is important to note that the fungal-mold on rancid walnuts produces aflatoxin, a potent carcinogen. A mold infested walnut seed batch should not be screened: but rather the entire batch should be discarded (thrown away).

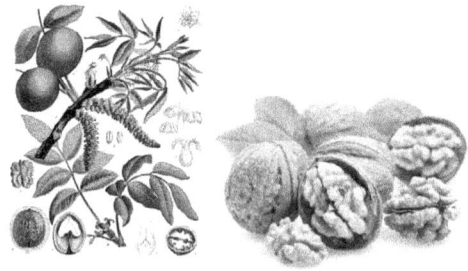

SUMMARY OF NUTS

Nuts, in general, are the best source of <u>arginine, an amino acid</u> that plays an important role in lowering blood pressure, <u>wound healing</u>, <u>detoxification</u>, <u>immune functioning</u>, preventing and/or treating erectile dysfunction as well as promoting the <u>secretion of several hormones, including insulin, sex hormones and growth hormones</u>.

Arginine supplementation has already been shown to be beneficial in a number of cardiovascular diseases, including angina pectoris, congestive heart failure, high blood pressure (this is because arginine has a relaxing effect on blood vessels), and peripheral vascular insufficiency (decreased blood flow to the legs or arms).

Arginine is needed in the formation of nitric oxide. Nitric oxide plays a central role in determining the tone of blood vessels. By increasing nitric oxide levels, arginine supplementation improves blood flow which is necessary for male sexual erections. <u>In fact, nitric oxide is the main component of Cialis, and Viagra</u>. Arginine also reduces blood clot formation, and improves blood fluidity. The benefits of arginine are attainable by eating foods high in arginine, such as nuts.

Interesting is the results of a recent study where it was found that the <u>people who consumed the most nuts were less obese</u>. A possible explanation is that nuts are high in fiber and low in carbohydrates and therefore <u>the consumption of nuts produces satiety</u>.

This same study demonstrated that higher nut consumption was associated with a protective effect against heart attacks. Other studies have linked the consumption of nuts to a reduced risk of heart disease, in general, and also lowered the risk of type 2 diabetes.

This link may be related to the phytonutrients in nuts and their ability to fix the damage (heal) done by high glucose and insulin levels in the blood as well as toxins and free radicals and therefore improve cell membrane structure and receptor function.

It is now well documented that abnormal or damaged cell membrane structures (i.e. insulin receptors) are due to eating the wrong types of foods (those that do not have enough anti-oxidants and anti-inflammatory nutrients for the amount of trans-fats and non-nutritive artificial sugars consumed).

Eating foods high in sugars and saturated fats, especially the hydrogenated oils or trans-fats are known to produce or cause free radical damage. And this damage to cell receptors leads to impaired action of insulin and LDL cholesterol, the bad cholesterol if oxidized by free radicals. Clinical studies have shown that increasing the intake of mono-unsaturated fats found in nuts and seeds improves insulin action and the production of HDL cholesterol, the good cholesterol. Still other studies have indicated that frequent consumption of olive oil, nuts and nut oils protects against the development of type 2 diabetes, even in subjects who are obese, even though obesity is a major risk factor for both cardiovascular diseases and type 2 diabetes.

Vegetable Oils

Nuts and seeds have long been used as a source of oils for culinary, medicinal, and cosmetic purposes. For culinary purposes, oils can be used in salad dressings and sauces, in baking and in cooking.

Some oils offer advantages over others for certain application. For example, olive oil, macadamia nut oil, coconut oil, sesame seed oil, and canola oil are more stable than other oils and are therefore preferred for use when exposing foods to heat.

It is important to make sure the cooking temperature does not go above the smoke point of these oils because they then become bad (oxidized) oils which produces a cascade of free radicals.

Canola oil and coconut oil has gained incredible popularity in a short period of time because it is being promoted for its high level of omega-3 fatty acids.

Other good oils, such as flaxseed, safflower, soy, and sunflower, are not recommended if they are going to be exposed to heat because the heat oxidizes (changes) the chemical structures of the fatty acids and forms free radicals.

These oils are good for culinary use, but only if the food does not have to be heated above 100 degrees Fahrenheit, i.e. use these oils in making salad dressings.

Other oils, such as margarine and shortening which are either trans-fatty acids (trans-fats), or partially hydrogenated oils (still a trans-fat), as well as cottonseed oil are best avoided altogether.

In fact, because cottonseed oil has demonstrated in men who had used the crude cottonseed oil as their cooking oil had low sperm counts followed by total testicular failure. Interesting though is: this oil is being investigated now as an anti-fertility agent or 'male birth control pill'.

Fish oil, flaxseed oil, evening primrose oil, borage oil, and black currant oils are mainly used for medicinal purposes. Black currant oil contains gamma-linolenic acid, an omega-6 fatty acid, which acts as a precursor of one of the favorable prostaglandins (an anti-inflammatory agent) for the treatment of arthritis and other inflammatory conditions.

Flaxseed oil may provide greater benefit due to it high concentration of linolenic acid, an omega-3 fatty acid. Flaxseed oil also contains linoleic acid, which is easily converted to gamma-linolenic acid by most people.

Fish oils are rich in eicosapentaenoic (EPA) and other omega-3 oils and are quite popular as medicinal agents for preventing and treating cardiovascular disease and other inflammatory disease. In fact, fish oil is well known for its anti-inflammatory properties and is known to prevent and/or reduce all metabolic age related medical diseases.

Selecting and Storing Nuts and Seeds

In general, nuts and seeds, due to their high oil content, are best purchased and stored in their shells. The shell is a natural protector against free-radical damage caused by oxidation which occurs naturally when exposed to light and air. Make sure the shells are free of splits, cracks, stains, holes, or other surface imperfections.

Do not eat or use moldy nuts or seeds, and also avoid limp, rubbery dark, or shriveled nutmeats. Store nuts and seeds within shells in a cool, dark, dry environment for up to two to three months. If you must buy shelled nuts or seeds, store them in air-tight containers in the refrigerator or freezer. *Crushed nuts, slivered nuts, and nut pieces that you may find for sale are the types most often rancid.*

Tips for Nut and Seed Preparation

In addition to being eaten as snacks, nuts and seeds can be added to many foods for their unique flavor. For instance, you can add ground walnuts to any cereal and the nutritional value and taste of that cereal will increase 4 fold. With the aid of a food processor, nut and seed butters can be prepared right at home.

Most nuts and seeds have enough natural oils to make nut butter. Keep nut butters in airtight containers in the refrigerator, where they will usually keep for three to six months.

You can also prepare your own, healthier version of dry-roasted nuts by laying them out on a baking sheet and then roasting them in an over at 275 degree (F) for 15 to 20 minutes.

Nuts and seeds, like grains and legumes, can be sprouted. Sprouting is thought to not only increase their nutritional value, but also improve their digestibility as well.

All you need to do for sprouting seeds and nuts at home is a large glass jar. After rinsing the nuts or seeds once or twice, cover with pure (non-chlorinated) water for 24 hours. After the initial 24 hours, pour out the water, rinse, and allow the moist nuts or seed to sprout in an area without direct sunlight. Rinse the nuts or seed twice daily.

Once the item has sprouted (usually in one to three days), it can be placed in more direct sunlight if desired. Most sprouts will be ready to eat one to two days after they have sprouted.

Omega 3 and Omega 6 Fatty Acids

There are two types of essential polyunsaturated fats. They are known as omega 3 fatty acid and omega 6 fatty acid: (omega-3 and omega-6).

Both of these are considered Essential Fatty Acids (EFA) because the human body cannot make either of them.

We get these healthy essential fatty acids from the foods we eat. For instance, Linoleic Acid (LA) is used by fish to make Alpha linolenic acid (ALA). Alpha Linolenic Acid (ALA) is the most common omega 3 fatty acid. Then ALA is used to make Eicosapentaenoic acid (EPA) which is the type of omega-3 fatty acid found in fish oils.

Note: Linoleic Acid (LA) is really an omega 6 fatty acid and is found in seed oils of vegetables and Alpha Linolenic Acid (ALA) is mainly found in leaves but some is found in seed oils.

Our body can make other fatty acids from excess calories we consume. One of these nonessential fatty acids is arachidonic acid is made by our body from the omega-6 fatty acid, i.e., Linoleic Acid (LA). Arachidonic Acid is a very important precursor of some very important powerful hormones known collectively as "eicosanoids".

Eicosanoids are signaling molecules made by oxidation of 20-carbon fatty acids. They exert complex control over many bodily systems, mainly in inflammation and/or immunity, as well as act as messengers in the central nervous system.

The networks of controls that depend upon eicosanoids are among the most complex in the human body. Eicosanoids are derived from either omega-3 or omega-6 fatty acids. The omega-6 eicosanoids are generally anti-inflammatory: omega-3s are much less so.

The amounts and balance of these fats in a person's diet will affect the body's eicosanoid-controlled functions, with effects on cardiovascular disease, triglycerides, blood pressure, and arthritis.

Essential Fatty Acids (Omega-3 fatty acid and Omega-6 fatty acid) are important because they are also needed by the body to build the phospholipids in the membranes that surround each cell. If there becomes a deficiency of these essential fatty acids (EPA) then the membranes become weak and allow diseases to form.

These "essential fatty acids" are also involved and needed for the transport LDL-cholesterol into the cells through receptors located in every cell's membrane. This is why it can be said that essential fatty acids like Omega-3 fatty acid can and do lower cholesterol from the blood.

Next, and very important for health, is the fact that eicosanoids (powerful hormones like prostaglandins, leukotrienes, and thromboxanes) are made from these essential fatty acids (omega-3s and omega-6s). When there is a deficiency of these essential fatty acids our body many different diseases and illnesses may occur.

For instance, our body may fail to thrive and skin problems like scaliness and increased water loss may occur. These skin disorders lose their protective ability against the intrusion of germs and chemicals and the body becomes more susceptible to infections. Other abnormalities caused by deficiencies of these essential fatty acids are weaknesses in the cardiovascular system and neurological system as well as kidney and fertility problems

Deficiency of these essential fatty acids occur most often in people who do not eat enough vegetables, seeds and nuts. **Depletion of essential fatty acid occurs more in today's world through the ingestion of hydrogenation of vegetable oils (trans-fats) that are found in margarine and shortening and the milling of grains where the bran and wheat germ (the healthy ingredients of grains) are removed by refining.**

Also, deficiencies of these essential fatty acids occur when we do not consume enough of the good omega-3 fatty acid foods, like fish and nuts and seeds and their oils in our daily diet.

Note: Deficiencies of essential fatty acids play a significant role in the formation of atherosclerosis, coronary thrombosis, multiple sclerosis, complications of diabetes mellitus, hypertension, and some forms of cancer.

Just by adding more foods that contain linoleic acid and alpha linoleic acid is known to correct or heal the diseases caused by the deficiency of these essential fatty acids. Studies indicate that the consumption of omega-3 fatty acids from fish and or fish oils (alpha linoleic acid) foods should be higher than the consumption of omega-6 fatty acid (linoleic acid) foods. However, the consumption of both of these essential fatty acids can prevent most of the chronic metabolic diseases that prevail in our modern day industrial world.

Hydrogenated Oils

Oils have been hydrogenated for many decades, only for the purpose of prolonging their shelf life and make the oils more stable. Hydrogenated oil is oil in which the essential fatty acids have been converted to a different form chemically, which has several effects.

Hydrogenated oil is far more shelf stable, and will not go rancid as quickly as untreated oil. It also has a higher melting point, and is often used in frying and pastries for this reason. When hydrogenated, the chemical structure of the oil is changed.

In the 1990s, it was realized that these products might have deleterious health effects, a tragic irony since these products, margarine and shortening, were originally produced and promoted as being healthier than conventional oils and fats.

Hydrogenated oil is made by forcing hydrogen gas into oil at high pressure. Both animal and vegetable fats can be and are hydrogenated. In general, the more solid the oil is, the more hydrogenated it is. Two common examples of hydrogenated oil are Crisco and margarine.

Note: if you were to heat up a stick of margarine in a very hot oven for over 2 hours you would end up with a glob of plastic! Also notice how margarine melts in a hot frying pan compared to natural butter or lard.

CHAPTER 6 HERBS AND SPICES

Plants play a major role in modern pharmaceuticals. Many modern drugs were initially derived from plants, and screening for medicinal plant compounds is still an important aspect of modern research. Generally, the practice is to find compounds that can be used as the base from which to develop a patentable medication. However, research is continuing to grow into the use of herbs as opposed to semi-synthetic medications designed to mimic the natural plant nutrient. Herbs are currently being raised commercially for this very purpose.

Technically, an herb is a plant that does not have a woody stem. If a plant has a woods stem, it is referred to as a shrub, bush or tree. The term "herb" is also used to describe a plant or plant part that is used for medicinal purposes. A "spice", on the other hand is technically a plant product that has aromatic properties and can be used medicinally and to season or flavor foods. Most spices are derived from bark, for example, cinnamon and nutmeg: or from dried fruits, for example, red and black pepper. Herbs used in cooking are typically composed of leaves and stems.

This explanation makes for an easy way to distinguish herbs from spices. **But just for the record, herbs can be spices and spices can be herbs.**

Herbs and spices make good sources of medicinal products. Many herbalists have used herbs and crude plant extracts as effective medicines for years. In fact, many pharmaceutical companies use the knowledge gained from herbalists to then isolate a particular part of that plant product as a drug and then market it as a medicine. For many people in the world, herbal medicines are the only therapeutic agents available. The World Health Organization has estimated that perhaps 80 percent of the world's population relies on traditional natural therapies.

It can be safely stated that the majority of the world's population relies on plants as medicines.

However, most people in the United States still know very little of the tremendous value of plants as medicine even though the rest of the world, especially in Europe and Asia, has experienced a tremendous renaissance in the use and appreciation of herbal medicine. Nonetheless, herbal teas and products are a major business in the United States as well, with an estimated annual sales figure of more than **$4 billion.**

This rebirth of herbal medicine, especially in developed countries, is largely based on renewed interest by the public and scientific researchers. During the last 20 to 30 years, there has been an explosion of scientific information concerning plants, crude plant extracts, and various substances from plants as medicinal agents. This research has lead to increased marketing and consumption of herbal remedies.

COMMONLY USED HERBS AND SPICES AND THEIR MEDICINAL VALUE

1. **Anise** (Pimpinella anisum) is a member of the Umbelliferae family along with celery, fennel, dill, and carrots as well as coriander, cumin, and caraway. Anise provides the stronger, true taste of licorice.

   The oils are distilled from the seeds to impart a strong licorice flavor to candies, cough syrups, alcoholic beverages, breath mints, etc. Anise provides similar benefits to those of fennel in that it is a rich source of cancer-preventing coumarin compounds, which are the primary components in anise's relatively high concentration of volatile oils.

   Anise is mildly estrogenic but much weaker than fennel. Together, the compounds in anise exert a broad range of health benefits, but primarily they help expel gas (carminative effect), relax intestinal spasms (antispasmodic effect), and relieve coughs (anti-tussive effect). Reportedly a few seeds taken with water will often cure hiccups.

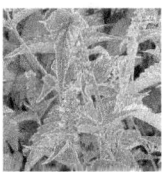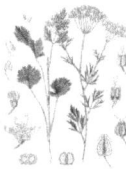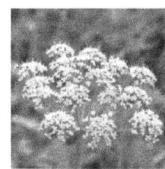

2. **Basil** (Ocimum basilicum) is a mint and belongs to the same family as peppermint. While the taste of sweet basil is sweet, there are other varieties that differ from this well-known taste, such as lemon basil, anise (licorice) basil, and cinnamon basil, which all have names indicative of their respective flavor variation. Basil has many of the same medicinal effects as other members of the mint family. Specifically it is used as

a <u>digestive aid</u>, as a <u>mild sedative</u> and for the <u>treatment of headaches</u>.

The herb is still used in China for spasms of the intestinal tract, kidney ailments, and poor circulation. The volatile oil of basil relaxes the smooth muscle of the intestines and <u>dilates small blood vessels</u>.

The volatile oil of a variety of sweet basil has been shown to possess antibacterial as well as anthelmintic (antiworm) activities, which would make it effective in treating the <u>intestinal ailments</u>.

Research studies on basil have shown it to contain orientin and vicenin, two water-soluble flavonoids that protect cell structures as well as chromosomes from radiation and free-radical damage. As such, basil provides important <u>anti-cancer properties</u>.

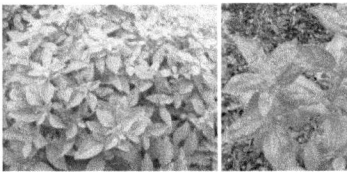

3.   **Bay leaf:** Also called laurel leaf or bay laurel. This aromatic herb comes from the evergreen bay laurel tree, native to the Mediterranean. Early Greeks and Romans attributed magical properties to the laurel leaf and it has long been a <u>symbol of honor</u>, <u>celebration and triumph</u>, as in "winning your laurels." The two main varieties of bay leaf are Turkish (which has 1- to 2-inch-long oval leaves) and Californian (with narrow, 2- to 3-inch-long leaves). The Turkish bay leaves have a more subtle flavor than do the California variety.

Bay leaves are used to flavor soups, stews, vegetables and meats. They're generally removed before serving. Overuse of this herb can make a dish bitter. Fresh bay leaves are seldom available in markets. Dried bay leaves, which have a fraction of the flavor of fresh, can be found in supermarkets. Store dried bay leaves airtight in a cool, dark place for up to 6 months.

 Bay leaves contain small amounts of vitamins. Vitamin A offers the most at 25 mg or 3 percent of the daily recommended intake for this vitamin. Trace amounts of vitamin B1, B2, B3, B6 and B9 (thiamine, riboflavin, niacin, pyridoxine and folate respectfully) are found in bay leaves. Bay leaves contain small amounts of dietary minerals, including iron, calcium and magnesium. Trace quantities of minerals are also found in bay leaves, including phosphorus, zinc and potassium.

4. **Cardamom** (Elettaria cardamomum) is a perennial plant with simple erect stems (or canes) that can reach a height of 10 feet. The small green fruit contains up to 18 seeds.

Cardamom tastes like an airy, gentle ginger with a touch of pine. Cardamom is used prominently in curry powder and it is also used in desserts, especially pastries, and as a fragrance in soaps, detergents, lotions and perfumes.

Cardamom's prime uses are similar to those of cinnamon and ginger – as a carminative, digestive aid, and stimulant. It is also a valuable flavoring agent for herbal medicinal preparations for indigestion and flatulence.

147

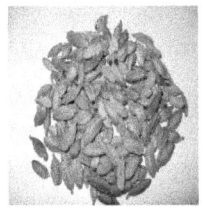 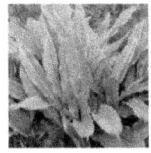 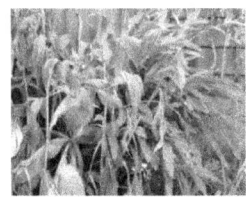

5. **Cayenne (red) Pepper and Paprika** (Capsicum frutenscens) is the fruit of Capsicum annuum longum, a shrubby tropical plant that can grow to a height of up to 3 feet. The fruit is technically a berry. Cayenne and most other Capsicum varieties are typically moderately to very spicy.

   However, paprika is a milder, sweeter-tasting fruit produced by a different variety of Capsicum annuum. Capsaicin is the main chemical with medicinal properties. This compound is well recognized in clinical research as an effective <u>pain reliever</u>: as a <u>digestive and antiulcer aid</u>: and for its <u>cardiovascular benefits</u>.

   Capsaicin is also the component responsible for cayenne pepper's **thermogenic** ability to <u>increase basal metabolic rate and stimulate the burning of fat for energy</u>. This is called (lipid oxidation or fat burning).

   In a recent study <u>the burning of fat</u> for energy was significantly enhanced by the addition of red pepper to either meal, but especially the high-fat meal. <u>Similar results have been noted with garlic and ginger</u>. The bottom line from this study and others is that adding red pepper as well as garlic and ginger to your diet is a safe, natural way to enhance the burning of fat.

Capsaicin-containing creams and gels are available as FDA-approved topical treatments for <u>arthritis</u> and <u>pain</u> relief such as that seen in <u>diabetic neuropathy</u>, <u>psoriasis</u>, <u>rheumatoid arthritis</u>, and <u>post- herpes pain</u> (post herpetic neuralgia).

Topical capsaicin preparations have been shown to be an effective treatment for <u>cluster headaches</u> and <u>osteoarthritis pain</u>.

Capsaicin also has a stimulating effect on the mucus membranes of the nose and sinuses. Capsaicin stimulates blood flow through the membranes and causes mucus secretions to become thinner and more liquid. This action makes it beneficial in relieving nasal congestion and combating the <u>common cold or sinus infection</u>.

Perhaps the most important internal benefit is its effects of stimulating and enhancing digestion. A recent study found that daily doses of red pepper significantly reduced symptoms of indigestion in individuals with frequent indigestion (functional dyspepsia).

It was found to reduce episodes of nausea, stomach pain, and stomach fullness. There is some evidence that spicy foods containing cayenne and turmeric may actually <u>help heal peptic ulcer</u>.

Also, cayenne pepper also exerts a number of beneficial effects on the <u>cardiovascular system</u>. Specifically, it reduces the likelihood of developing atherosclerosis by reducing blood cholesterol and triglyceride levels and platelet aggregation as well as increasing fibrinolytic activity. Fibrinolytic activity refers to the ability to prevent the formation of blood clots, which can lead to a heart attack, stroke, or pulmonary embolism.

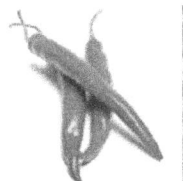 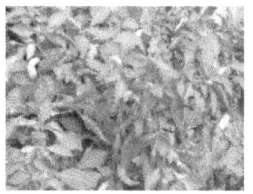 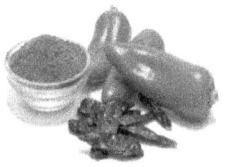

6. **Chia: Salvia hispanica or Salvia columbariae**, are species of flowering plants in the <u>mint</u> family, Lamiaceae. The seeds can be ground or used whole for nutritious drinks and as a food source.

 Chia is an **<u>annual herb</u>** growing to (3.3 ft) tall, with opposite leaves. Its flowers are purple or white and are produced in numerous clusters in a spike at the end of each stem. Many plants cultivated as S. hispanica are actually S. lavandulifolia.

Chia is grown commercially for its seed, a food that is rich in <u>omega-3 fatty acids</u>, since the seeds include <u>α-linolenic acid (ALA)</u>. Chia seeds are typically small ovals with a diameter of about (0.04 in). They are mottle-colored with brown, gray, black and white.

Today, chia (salvia hispanica) is grown commercially in its native Mexico, as well as in Bolivia, Argentina, Ecuador, Australia, and Guatemala. A one ounce serving of chia seeds contains 9 grams of fat (80 calories), sodium, dietary fiber and protein.

 Chia seeds also have calcium, phosphorus and manganese, which are similar in nutrient content to other edible seeds such as flax or sesame. Research indicates chia has a great potential for <u>dietary health benefits</u>. Chia seed consumption has been reported in the public media and is purportedly used by athletes.

Chia Seed is known as a "super" food that can fit into any diet.

This seed has tremendous nutritional value and medicinal properties. For centuries this tiny little seed was used as a staple food by the Indians of the south west and Mexico.

Known as the running food, its use as a high energy endurance food has been recorded as far back as the ancient Aztecs. It was said the Aztec warriors subsisted on the Chia seed during the conquests. The Indians of the south west would eat as little as a teaspoon full when going on a 24hr. forced march.

Chia seeds may be added to other foods as a topping or put into smoothies, oatmeal, yogurt, made into a gelatin substance, or consumed raw. Because there is no perceptible shell, addition of chia seeds to other products may not alter taste.

 Interesting and useful to note is the fact that if you try mixing a spoonful of Chia in a glass of water and leaving it for approximately 30 minutes or so, when you return the glass will appear to contain not seeds or water, but an almost solid gelatin.

This gel-forming reaction is due to the soluble fiber in the Chia. Researchers believe this same gel-forming phenomenon takes place in the stomach when food containing these gummy fibers, known as mucilages, are eaten.

The gel that is formed in the stomach creates a physical barrier between carbohydrates and the digestive enzymes that break them down, thus slowing the conversion of carbohydrates into sugar. This slowing in the conversion of carbohydrates into sugar offers the ability for creating endurance and has obvious benefits for diabetics.

Carbohydrates are the fuel for energy in our bodies. Prolonging their conversion into sugar stabilizes metabolic changes, diminishing the surges of highs and lows in level of blood insulin thus creating a longer duration in the fueling effects of carbohydrates.

Because there is a greater efficiency in the utilization of body fluids with chia seeds, the electrolyte balance is maintained. This is because the Chia seed has hydrophilic properties, and has the ability to absorb more than 12 times its weigh in water. Its ability to hold on to water offers the ability to prolong hydration.

Fluids and electrolytes provide the environment that supports the life of all the body's cells. Their concentration and composition are regulated to remain as constant as possible.

With Chia seeds, you retain moisture, regulate, more efficiently, the body's absorption of nutrients and body fluids.

 Note: Chia (salvia hispanica) is the main ingredient in the Aztec weight loss diet.

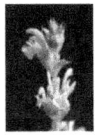 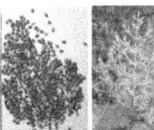

7. **Chives** belong to the same family as <u>onions</u> (Allium): the lily family and therefore have the same nutritional and health benefits as onions.

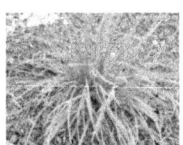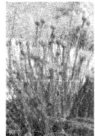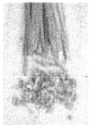

8. **Cinnamon** (Cinnamomum verum) comes from the inner bark of evergreen trees native to southwest India and Asia. In addition to its use as a spice, cinnamon or its oil is used as a flavoring agent in pharmaceutical, personal health, and cosmetic products.

Cinnamon has a long history of use in both Eastern and Western cultures as a medicine. Some of its reported uses are in cases of <u>arthritis</u>, <u>asthma</u>, <u>cancer</u>, <u>diarrhea</u>, <u>fever</u>, <u>heart problems</u>, <u>diabetes</u>, <u>insomnia</u>, <u>menstrual problems</u>, <u>peptic ulcers</u> <u>psoriasis</u> and <u>spastic muscles</u>.

Cinnamon's unique healing abilities come from three basic components in the essential oils found in its bark. These oils contain active components called cinnamaldehyde, cinnamyl acetate, and cinnamul alcohol, plus a wide range of other volatile substances. There are several multi-component herbal formulas in use to treat <u>epilepsy</u>, <u>common cold</u>, <u>influenza</u>.

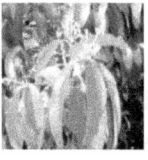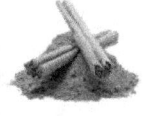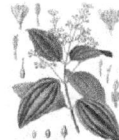

9. **Cloves** come from the unopened flower bud of the clove tree. The flesh of the clove features an oily compound (oil of cloves) that is essential to their medicinal, nutritional, and gustatory profile.

Cloves have a warm, sweet, and aromatic taste that evokes the sultry tropical climates where they are grown. Cloves are native to the Moluccas, which is an Indonesian group of volcanic islands formerly known as the Spice Islands.

Cloves contain significant amounts of an active nutrient called eugenol, which has made them the subject of numerous health studies, including studies showing benefit for the prevention of toxicity from environmental pollutants, such as carbon tetrachloride: prevention of digestive tract cancers: and treatment of joint inflammation. Eugenol can be used as a dental anesthetic as well as an antiseptic.

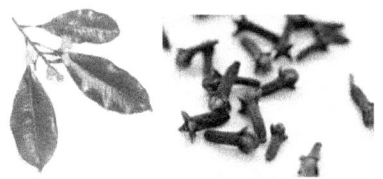

10. **Coriander** (**Cilantro**) is a bright green annual with slender, erect hollow stems. (Coriandrum sativum) is considered both an herb and a spice, since both its leaves and its dried ripe fruits, which are known as coriander seeds. These are used as a seasoning condiment. Fresh coriander leaves are well known as **cilantro**, and they bear a strong likeness to the Italian flat-leaf parsley, both of which belong to the Umbelliferae family.

Coriander seeds have a health-supporting reputation that is high on the list of the healing spices. The essential oils in the seed make it an effective carminative and digestive aid. In parts of Europe, coriander has traditionally been referred to as an <u>anti-diabetic plant</u>. In parts of India, it has traditionally been used for its <u>anti-inflammatory</u> properties (arthritis and/or swelling).

Modern scientific investigations of coriander have focused on its <u>anti-microbial </u>properties, <u>anti-anxiety</u> action and <u>cholesterol-lowering</u> action is the result of coriander stimulating the conversion of cholesterol to bile acids within the liver, an effect that would likely improve digestion of fat.

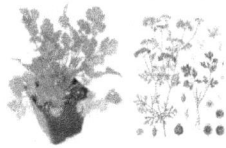

11. **Cumin** (Cuminum cyminum) possesses a powerful flavor described as being peppery, mustard like with slight citrus overtones. Cumin is the dried seed of the herb Cuminum cyminum, a member of the <u>parsley family</u>. <u>Cumin seeds</u> have been noted to be of benefit to the digestive system. This spice probably does this by stimulating the secretion of pancreatic enzymes, important factors in proper digestion and nutrient assimilation.

As with other carminative spices, cumin's digestive stimulating effects are due to its content of volatile oils. Cumin seeds may also have <u>anti-cancer properties</u>. This cancer-protective effect may be due to cumin's potent free-radical scavenging abilities, as well as the ability it has shown to <u>enhance the liver's detoxification enzymes</u>.

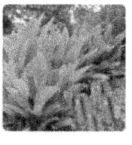 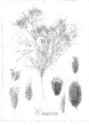

12. **Dill** (Anethum graveolens) is a member of the Umbelliferae family along with carrot, celery, fennel, and parsley. Dill's prime health benefit is similar to that of other aromatic herbs, As a carminative it aids in the elimination of flatulence and digestive disturbance. Like other aromatic herbs, dill (dill seed) has shown some anti-cancer and antimicrobial effects.

The two major classes of active compounds in dill are the monoterpenes in the volatile oil: including carvone, limonene and anethofuran, and unique flavonoids. Dill is especially useful in promoting detoxification reactions in the liver to help the liver rid the body of toxic chemical. The monoterpene components of dill have been shown to activate the liver enzyme helps attach the antioxidant molecule glutathione-S-tranferase.

This enzyme helps attach the antioxidant molecule glutathione to toxic molecules that would otherwise do damage in the body. This action makes dill a "chemoprotective" food that can help neutralize particular types of carcinogens, such as the benzopyrenes that are part of cigarette smoke, charcoal grill smoke and the smoke produced by trash incinerators.

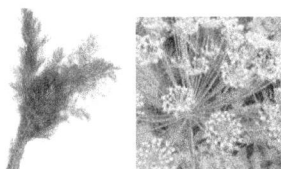

13. **Garlic** is considered to be both a vegetable and an herb. It is a species in the onion genus, Allium. Its close relatives include the onion, shallot, leek, and chive. The garlic plant's bulb is the most commonly used part of the plant. With the

exception of the single clove types, garlic bulbs are normally divided into numerous fleshy sections called cloves.

Garlic cloves are used for consumption (raw or cooked) as a nutrient for taste and for medicinal purposes. Garlic is increasingly being used for medicinal purposes in order to prevent or treat many diseases and health conditions.

Garlic has been shown to play a beneficial role in lowering your cholesterol levels and therefore reducing the hardening of arteries and the development of heart disease. It probably does this by reducing the formation of cholesterol by liver cells much like the statin drugs.

Research has indicated that a high intake of garlic protects against the development of colorectal and gastric cancers. This effect has not been verified in other types of cancer. If you have high blood pressure, taking garlic may help you reduce your levels to a healthier range.

Studies indicate garlic can reduce blood pressure both in people with high blood pressure and those with normal blood pressure. Consuming garlic has been known to be a form of treatment for certain fungal infections of your skin, including ringworm, athlete's foot and jock itch.

 You can just apply garlic gel to the skin and have a positive impact on relieving these infections. Note: You can boost your intake of garlic with garlic cloves, garlic tablets or garlic capsules.

Garlic may be applied to different kinds of bread to create a variety of classic dishes, such as garlic bread, garlic toast, bruschetta, crostini and canapé. Oils can be flavored with garlic cloves. These infused oils are used to season all categories of vegetables, meats, breads and pasta.

In some cuisines, the young bulbs are pickled for three to six weeks in a mixture of sugar, salt, and spices. Scrapes generally have a milder taste than the cloves. They are often used in stir frying or braised like asparagus.

Garlic leaves are a popular vegetable in many parts of Asia. The leaves are cut, cleaned, and then stir-fried with eggs, meat, or vegetables. Mixing garlic with egg yolks and olive oil produces aioli. Garlic, oil, and a chunky base produce skordalia. Blending garlic, almond, oil, and soaked bread produces ajoblanco. Garlic powder has a different taste from fresh garlic. Note: If used as a substitute for fresh garlic, 1/8 teaspoon of garlic powder is equivalent to one clove of garlic.

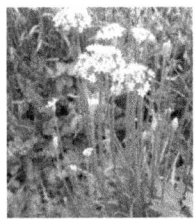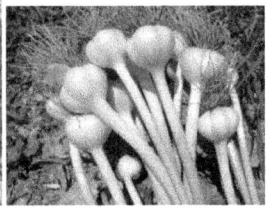

14. **Ginger** (Zingiber officinale) is an erect perennial herb that has thick tuberous rhizomes (underground roots). Ginger is a herb but is also considered and known as a spice, with a strong distinct flavor that can increase the production of saliva. The part that is used as spice on the plant itself is the rhizomes or ginger root.

    Cooking Info: This ginger root is traditionally used with sweet foods in Western cuisine being included in popular recipes such as ginger ale, ginger snaps, gingerbread, ginger biscuits and ginger cake. It is also used in many countries as a medicinal ingredient which many believe in.

Medicinal Info: Ginger is known to help cure diabetes, headaches, colds, fatigue, nausea and the flu when used in tea or food.

Ginger is known to promote <u>energy producing processes</u> in the body while positively <u>increasing the body's metabolic rate</u>.

The following is a list of **medicinal properties ginger** has been known to have throughout history: Antiemetic/anti-nausea, Anti-clotting agent, Antispasmodic, Antifungal, Anti inflammatory, Antiseptic, Antibacterial, Antiviral, Antitussive, Analgesic, Circulatory stimulant, Carminative, Expectorant, Hypotensive, Increases blood flow, Promotes sweating and Relaxes peripheral blood vessels.

Ginger is good for your health and has been said by some to be a plant directly from the Garden of Eden. It is also said that consuming Ginger before taking a plane flight can prevent motion sickness. It can make good tea.

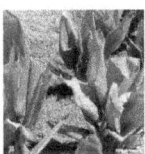 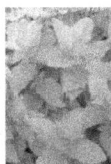 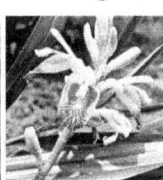 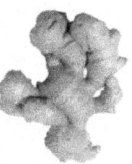

15. Horseradish: (Armoracia rusticana) is a perennial plant of the Brassicaceae family (which also includes mustard, wasabi, broccoli, and cabbage). The root of the horseradish plant can be eaten raw or used to create horseradish sauce. The leaves are edible and have some of the medicinal properties of the roots.

This plant is considered an herb. It is resistant to the low temperatures as well as to droughts and grows in the shaded places as well as the warm places. It does not grow well in sandy soils but it does grow well in clay-like alkaline soils rich in humus.

Horseradish can be used throughout the year in preparing various meal recipes and because of its spicy flavor the horseradish root can be used in conserving the canned food for the winter.

Horseradish is used in marinades and as an accompaniment to meats. Its sharp, pungent, spicy flavor can provide a unique flavor contrast. But horseradish also provides significant *nutritional properties:* One tablespoon of prepared horseradish contains about seven (7) calories. The horseradish contains virtually no saturated fat and no cholesterol. They contain dietary fiber, some sugars, protein, a nutrient your body uses to repair itself after injury or exercise. vitamin C, folate, potassium, calcium.

Horseradish is one of the richest foods in glucosinolates available. Glucosinolates are a type of glucose-containing compound that can help prevent the appearance of new tumors and fight the growth of existing tumors. The glucosinolates in horseradish can also contribute to the elimination of free radicals, therefore reducing your risk of cancer and other health conditions.

Medicinal properties: It has thick pulpy yellowy roots, spicy taste and antibiotic, anti-inflammatory and aphrodisiacal (a substance that increases sexual desire) properties. As a medicine, horseradish root has many curative properties: i.e., strong antibiotic, expectorant, bronchodilatator, antibacterial, coronary vasodilatator, it increases the blood pressure, it heats up the body, stimulates the body's immune system, anti-inflammatory, anti-parasitic, anti-anemic, antiscorbutic, and diuretic. It can stimulate the appetite. It has a cardiotonic effect and is recommended to the people that suffer from high blood pressure.

Also it is known that horseradish has aphrodisiacal (sexual arousal) properties. Some of the medical conditions that horseradish will help prevent or cure are: bronchitis, sinusitis, rheumatism, anemia, flu, stomatitis, and even facial paralysis can be treated by using horseradish.

As a treatment for sinusitis and rhinitis, just place a cataplasm (a warm moist preparation placed on an aching or inflamed part of the body to ease pain, improve circulation, or hasten the expression of pus) on the forehead along with two spoons of grained horseradish so that the nose gets immediately decongested. This treatment may be repeated 4 to 5 days in a row and it gets interrupted once burns occur.

As a treatment for bronchitis, flu and lung congestions, you may use horseradish flour and apply it like a cataplasm on the chest area for a half an hour up to an hour. This treatment may be repeated once every two or three days.

The pains caused by rheumatism can be treated in a similar manner using a cataplasm of horseradish over the painful inflamed area. If a burning sensation appears the treatment is to be stopped.

Gargling tincture of horseradish alleviates stomatitis. (*Stomatitis is an inflammation of the mucous lining of any of the structures in the mouth, which may involve the cheeks, gums, tongue, lips, throat, and roof or floor of the mouth. The inflammation can be caused by conditions in the mouth itself, such as poor oral hygiene, dietary protein deficiency, poorly fitted dentures, or from mouth burns and scars from food or drinks, toxic plants, or by conditions that affect the entire body, such as medications, allergic reactions, radiation therapy, or infections).* Just rinse your mouth (affected area) with 3-4 spoons in a glass half filled with water.

And against paradontosis (paradontosis is a chronic disease of gums and ligaments teeth in the bone base that is characterized by bleeding gums) can chew grained horseradish or buy a toothpaste that has this mixture as an ingredient. Note: This herb is great for gums because of its strong stimulating effects.

As a treatment for asthma, bronchitis, breathing disorders, horseradish syrup is recommended. Horseradish mixtures can be in the form of: tinctures, horseradish vinegar, and horseradish flour or horseradish cataplasm.

The tincture of horseradish is prepared by graining horseradish and putting this in a glass vessel filled with alimentary alcohol and is left to mix for 8 days, after which the whole mixture is strained.

Horseradish syrup is obtained in the following way: grained horseradish root is mixed with 4 spoons of honey and are left to mix for several minutes. The mixture is strained and pressed with gauze. The raw syrup is obtained. The remains from the gauze are set to boil in a small quantity of water. After boiling, the mixture gets strained and then left to cool off, after which it gets mixed with the raw syrup. It is consumed by taking 3 spoons of the mixture a day.

Horseradish flour is prepared from the horseradish root that is cut into tiny squares and left near a heated stove to dry. After that they can be ground into grain. The whitish powder, called horseradish flour, can be stored, however with the passing of the time it loses some of its characteristics.

Horseradish vinegar can be made by filling a bottle with grained horseradish over which apple vinegar is poured until it gets filled to the top. This mixture, horseradish vinegar, can be consumed in small quantities to treat the abovementioned illnesses.

Warning, If you suffer from gastric ulcer, goiterous, thyroid, problems or renal (kidney) diseases, the consumption of horseradish is not advised.

Also, note, the consumption of horseradish is forbidden to children younger than 4 years old.

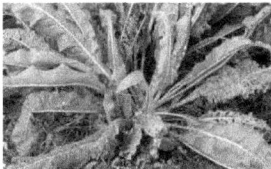 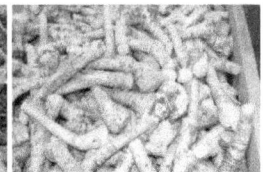

16. Marjoram and Oregano: Marjoram and Oregano are members of the mint family, Lamiaceae, considered the twin of thyme.

Marjoram has a more mild sweet flavor than oregano with perhaps a hint of balsam. It is said to be "the meat herb" that compliments all foods except sweets.

Marjoram, *Origunum marjorana*, is easy to grow from seed as long as you wait to plant until after all danger of frost has passed. It thrives with full sun and somewhat dry conditions, growing to a compact 8 or 10-inches. Mid-season, tiny white or pink clumps of flowers will form at the tips of the marjoram plant. To extend the life of the plant and encourage more leaf production, remove these buds as they form.

Although classified as a perennial, marjoram is sensitive to cold weather and will wither when exposed to frost. To bring it indoors for the winter, take clippings to root in water. In the warmest of climates, you may get another round of growth by cutting the plant back hard in the fall.

The delicate floral aroma of marjoram lends itself well to soaps, pomanders and herbal wreaths. Ornamental varieties such as the variegated or creeping types make attractive additions to the garden but are less flavorful than true sweet marjoram. Dried, the herb holds its lovely fragrance and its flavor much better than most other herbs do when dried.

Marjoram tea has been used historically for relief of symptoms from hay fever, sinus congestion, indigestion, asthma, stomach pain, headache, dizziness, colds, coughs, and nervous disorders. It is a gently fragrant, calming herb that does have mild antioxidant and anti-fungal properties.

Unsweetened tea can also be used as a mouthwash or gargle. Just take 1-2 cups of tea per day for the therapeutic benefits. Externally, marjoram leaves can be ground into a paste (if desired, hot tea or water, and a little oatmeal can be added for consistency purposes,), and used for the pain of rheumatism and for sprains. The leaves can be made into oil and used for relief of toothache pain. Just drop a few drops of the oil on the affected tooth. Leaves can also be placed in cheesecloth or a coffee filter and placed under the tap for a fragrant and refreshing bath that is believed good for the skin.

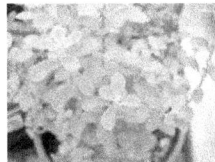 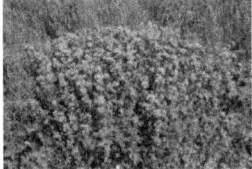

17. <u>Mint</u>: belongs to the mint family, Lamiaceae. It is an herb with remarkable medicinal properties. It is a well known mouth and breath freshener scientifically known as Mentha. The market is full of products containing mint ingredients - tooth paste, chewing gums, mouth & breath fresheners, candies and inhalers and even medicines, etc. which are based on mint.

Medicinal properties: Mint is not only a good appetizer but promotes digestion, due to its typical mint aroma. It also soothes the stomach in cases of <u>indigestion</u>, <u>nausea</u> and <u>inflammation</u>. This aroma of mint activates the saliva glands in our mouth as well as glands which secrete digestive enzymes, thereby facilitating digestion.

Medicinally it is used in medicines as the strong and refreshing aroma of mint is an excellent and quick remedy for nausea. Whenever you feel sick or nauseated, just <u>smell</u> the oil of mint or <u>crush</u> fresh mint leaves or use any product with mint flavor, i.e. mint tea, whichever is available near you, and nausea will be gone.

Balms based on mint or simply mint oil, when rubbed on forehead and nose, give quick <u>relief of a headache</u>. Respiratory Disorders like <u>sinus congestion</u>, <u>sore throat</u> and <u>cough</u> can be cured with mint products. The strong aroma of mint is very effective in opening up congestion of nose, throat, bronchi and lungs, <u>giving relief in respiratory disorders</u> resulting from asthma, cold, cough, etc.

As it cools and soothes throat, nose and other respiratory channels, it then relieves the cough too. Many balms are based on this property of mint. Unlike other inhalers which are

based on aerosols, those based on mint are more effective and eco-friendly too. Regular use of mint is very beneficial for asthma patients, as it is a <u>good smooth muscle relaxant</u> and gives <u>relief of congestion</u>.

While mint oil is a good <u>anti septic</u> and <u>anti pruritic</u>, mint juice is an excellent <u>skin cleanser</u>. It soothes skin, cures infections and itching and is also good for <u>removing pimples</u>.

Its anti pruritic properties can be used for treating bites of insects like mosquitoes, honey-bees, hornets, wasps, gnats etc. Being a germicidal and breath freshener, it takes care of oral health by inhibiting harmful bacterial growth inside mouth and by cleaning tongue and teeth.

Current research shows that certain enzymes present in mint may help cure cancer. Besides its wide industrial use in food stuffs such as ice-creams, chocolates etc., alcoholic and non-alcoholic beverages, cosmetics, medicines, inhalers and mouth and breathe fresheners, it is used as a condiment and decorative item in culinary world-wide.

Drinks and food-stuffs containing mint cool you off in summer. It is a good relaxant. One more peculiar property: it induces sweating if consumed in fever, thereby relieving fevers. <u>Mint juice can be applied on burns to heal and soothe them. It is beneficial in rheumatism.</u> It is also said to improve brain activity, although there are no sufficient proofs of this claim.

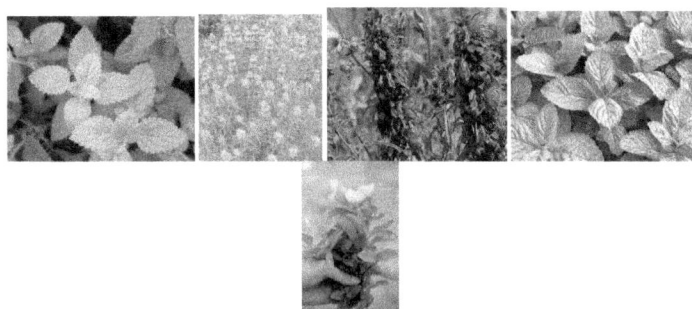

18. Mustard seeds: Mustard greens and mustard seeds are both a vegetable and an herb from the Brassica family. They are among the oldest known herbal remedies for a great number of health conditions.

There are three most commonly used types of mustard seeds, including brown mustard (Brassica juncea), white mustard (Brassica alba) and black mustard (Brassica nigra), which are available in powdered form or whole seeds.

Mustard seeds are used for producing oil, which is known for its excellent warming properties and can be used for massages. In addition, mustard seeds have very high nutritional value, being a source of many important microelements and nutrients.

One of the healthiest and the least caloric spices, mustard seeds are used in almost every world's cuisines and are among the world's most demanded spices.

Medicinal properties: Mustard seed benefits include anti-cancer and anti-inflammatory properties. Mustard seeds are a great source of selenium and magnesium, that are known to decrease inflammation and reduce the symptoms of such diseases as rheumatoid arthritis or asthma.

The seeds also contain isothiocyanates, known for their anti-cancer effects. Other useful elements and nutrients which can be found in mustard seeds and mustard greens are calcium, iron, manganese, phosphorus, zinc, niacin, dietary fiber and very valuable omega 3 fatty acids, which can lower cholesterol levels and protect us from having heart disease.

Since ancient times purgative properties were considered the best mustard seed benefits, but nowadays this herbal remedy is valued also for its antifungal and antiseptic effects. Mustard products have been used also to speed up metabolism and this way to improve the function of digestive system. One of the most important *health benefits* of mustard seeds is being helpful in reducing the frequency of <u>migraines</u>.

Mustard products and mustard oil have been effectively used for centuries for lowering <u>high blood pressure and preventing atherosclerosis</u>. Massaging your scalp with mustard oil will help you to substantially improve your hair quality and prevent hair loss.

Another interesting property of mustard seeds and mustard green is stimulating salivation and improving appetite. Finally, <u>mustard seed products can also help improve your immunity and assist in fighting against insomnia, as well to treat such problems as anxiety, psychological disorders, the effects of stresses and depression, bronchitis, sexual dysfunctions, the symptoms of menopause, and many others.</u>

(*An interesting note is that mustard seeds are the small round seeds of various mustard plants. The seeds are usually about 1 or 2 mm in diameter. Mustard seeds may be colored from yellowish white to black. They are important spices in many regional foods. The seeds can come from three different plants: black mustard (Brassica nigra), brown Indian mustard (B. juncea), and white mustard. B. hirta is the major species grown for seeds used in condiments. B. juncea and B. rapa var perviridis are most commonly grown for greens. The seeds of these greens will not hurt you, but will not have the flavor of the B. hirta species*).

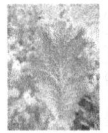 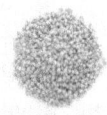 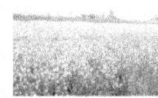

19. Nutmeg and Mace: Nutmeg and mace are two spices that come from the nutmeg tree. This tree is in the genus Myristica. The most important commercial species is Myristica fragrans, an evergreen tree indigenous to the Banda Islands (the Spice Islands) of Indonesia.

Nutmeg is not only known as a popular spice around the world, it is also popular for its many *health benefits*. Nutmeg can prevent and/or treat the following health problems. It can help eliminate and/or reduce fatigue, stress, symptoms of anxiety or depression, Nutmeg is also known to improve concentration.

Nutmeg is known to help relieve aching joints, muscle pain, arthritis, and other inflammatory problems. To relieve the pain, apply nutmeg oil to the affected areas. Nutmeg can effectively help relieve digestion-related problems like diarrhea, constipation, bloating, flatulence, etc.

Nutmeg oil can not only relieve stomachaches by removing the excess gas from your intestines, it can also boost your appetite. Because of its antibacterial properties, nutmeg can effectively treat halitosis or bad breath because of its antibacterial properties. Note: Bad breath is usually caused by a build-up of bacteria in your mouth and nutmeg can destroy these bacteria. For this reason, nutmeg is a common ingredient in many brands of toothpastes. Nutmeg, like horseradish, can also be used to treat gum problems and toothaches.

Detoxification is an important factor for good health. Because the liver and kidney are two of the organs that clean the blood of toxins. They are also the two organs where toxins build up and therefore need to be involved in detoxification. Nutmeg is a cleansing tonic: nutmeg can clean your liver and kidney and remove these toxins. Nutmeg is also effective in preventing and dissolving kidney stones. When your liver and kidney are successfully detoxified, they can perform their function better.

Nutmeg can actually help you achieve smoother and healthier skin by helping you treat several skin problems. For instance, a scrub made from nutmeg powder and orange lentil powder can help remove blackheads.

Nutmeg can also help make scars less noticeable. To help erase acne scars, just mix some nutmeg powder with some honey to make a paste, and then apply this mixture to the acne marks.

Drinking a cup of milk with some nutmeg powder will help you relax and induce sleep. **Mace** is a spice made from the waxy red covering that surrounds nutmeg seeds. The flavor is similar to that of nutmeg. Mace has a wide range of uses from desserts to savory roast meats. The versatile flavor can make mace a useful spice to have around, especially since many recipes call for it. Mace also has many of the medicinal properties of nutmeg and can be used in place of nutmeg to accomplish the same benefits.

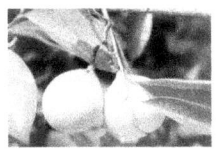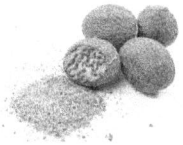

20. Oregano and Marjoram: Oregano belongs to the Origanum genus and the Lamiaceae family (mint family like marjoram). Even though oregano does not look particularly like marjoram, oregano but does have many of the same nutritional and medicinal properties. Marjoram has a more mild, sweet flavor than oregano with perhaps a hint of balsam.

Both are considered good for flavoring meats. Oil of oregano is promoted as a <u>potent purifier</u> that offers a long list of health *benefits*. The oil is made from the leaves and flowers of the oregano plant. *Medicinal qualities*. <u>Oregano oil</u> is an effective as an <u>antiviral</u>, an <u>antibacterial</u>, an <u>antifungal</u> and an <u>anti-parasitic</u> agent.

Oregano can also <u>diminish pain and inflammation</u> and cure certain infections. When applied directly to the skin, oil of oregano is said to have remedial effects on itchy or infected skin. Oregano oil is sometimes used in combination with olive oil or coconut oil. Diluted oregano is asserted to be a treatment for irritated gum tissue. Also, oregano can relieve symptom of sinus congestion, colds and viral infections.

Oregano oil is considered to be a natural treatment for sinus or lung congestion, sore throats, colds, stomach upset and mild indigestion. Research indicates that Oregano oil can offer protection against viral infections such as measles and mumps.

Oregano oil is also advertised as an antioxidant that protects the body from free radical damage.

<u>Oregano oils are very important as they have the ability to neutralize free radicals and slow down the aging process by helping to fight not only wrinkles but also vision and hearing loss</u> as well as <u>nervous disorders</u> such as <u>Alzheimer's disease and parkinsonism</u>.

The antioxidant effects of oregano are believed to also offer anti-aging benefits and protection against some cancers.

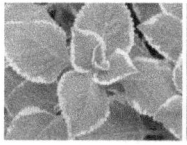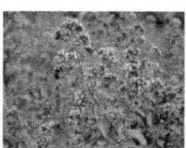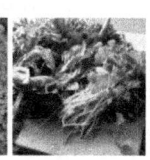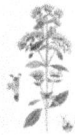

21. Rosemary: (Rosmarinus officinalis), commonly known as rosemary, is a woody, perennial herb with fragrant, evergreen, needle-like leaves and white, pink, purple, or blue flowers. It is a member of the mint family Lamiaceae, which includes many other herbs such as basil, lavender, myrtle, and sage.

Medicinal properties: Rosemary has strong antioxidant and muscle relaxant properties. Some healing benefits include the prevention of food poisoning, assists in infection prevention, relaxes the smooth muscle linings of both the uterus and stomach, and can act as a nasal decongestant. It also smells pretty good too.

Rosemary is very popular in the Mediterranean region as a culinary herb. Many dishes are cooked with rosemary oil and freshly plucked rosemary leaves. Rosemary essential oil is mostly extracted from the leaves.

Rosemary has been extensively used since ancient times for a variety of purposes. The Romans gave special importance to rosemary plant and used it in religious ceremonies. Its use extended to wedding ceremonies, food, cosmetics, and herbal care.

Rosemary plant and its extract were also used in the ancient Egyptian civilization as incense. The medicinal properties of rosemary essential oil are due to its ability to strengthen the entire body. Rosemary oil is thought to have the ability to detoxify and heal delicate organs such as liver, brain as well as heart.

Today, many medicinal preparations contain rosemary oil. Rosemary is known to relieve indigestion, flatulence and stomach cramps.

Rosemary leaves are often added to meat dishes as it helps in digesting meat, especially lamb, beef and pork.

Rosemary oil and rosemary teas are used extensively for hair care in shampoos and lotions. Regular use of rosemary oil helps in stimulating follicles, as a result, hair grows longer and stronger. It is also believed that rosemary oil slows down premature hair loss and graying of hair. Hence it is an excellent tonic for bald people.

Rosemary essential oil is also beneficial for dry and flaky scalps. Regular massage of scalp with rosemary oil nourishes the scalp and removes dandruff. Further, it is often mixed with tea tree oil and basil oil to treat scalp problems.

Rosemary essential oil is a disinfectant and can be used as a mouth wash. It also helps in removing bad breath much like other mints and horseradish. Rosemary essential oil can help in toning skin and removing dryness. It is also considered as a beauty aid for the face.

Rosemary essential oil, much like other mint oils and nutmeg oil are known as excellent brain and nerve tonics. They are often used by students during exam times as it increases concentration and helps in studying efficiently. These oils stimulate mental activity and relieve depression, mental fatigue and forgetfulness. Inhaling rosemary oil lifts your spirits immediately. Whenever your brain is tired, inhale rosemary oil to remove boredom and get fresh mental energy. The ability of rosemary essential oil to relieve pain has resulted in its extensive usage in headaches, muscle pains, sore muscles, rheumatism and even arthritis. Massaging the part which is in pain with rosemary essential oil can give relief from the pain.

Vapor baths with rosemary oil is found to be effective for rheumatism.

Rosemary has a mesmerizing aroma and hence rosemary essential oil is an excellent inhalant. The oil is used in room fresheners, cosmetics, beauty aids, food, bath oil, candles and perfumes due to its aroma. The oil, when inhaled brings mental energy and also clears the respiratory tract.

Many people spray mixture of rosemary essential oil and water to remove bad odor from room. The benefits of rosemary essential oil in treating respiratory problems are unmatched.

The scent of the oil gives relief from throat congestion, allergies, cold, sore throat and flu. Since rosemary oil is antiseptic it is effective for respiratory infections as well. The oil is antispasmodic and can be used in bronchial asthma.

Rosemary oil can help relieve menstrual cramps, peptic ulcer, urine flow, prostate, gall bladder, intestine, liver, cataract, heart, sperm mobility, leukemia, kidney stones and associated pain.

Research is also being carried out to study its potential in treating various types of cancers including colon cancer, stomach cancer, breast cancer, and lung cancer.

Since rosemary oil is volatile in nature, the oil may cause vomiting and spasms. It is suggested that rosemary essential oil should not be used by pregnant and breastfeeding or nursing women. Excessive dosage of the oil may lead to miscarriage or may affect the fetus.

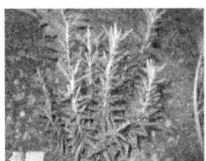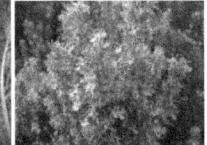

22. **Saffron**: is a spice derived from the flower of Crocus sativus, commonly known as the saffron crocus. Crocus is a genus in the family Iridaceae.

Saffron has been used as spice and coloring agent for many centuries and has numerous medicinal properties. Saffron is also used in many other industries such as the tobacco industry, alcohol industry, dairy industry, cosmetic industry for perfumes and facial creams, and the dye industry.

Hippocrates, and others attributed saffron with medical properties, because it is known to enhance digestion and strengthens the function of the stomach. Saffron can be used as a sedative. It can also be used to combats cough and cold symptoms. It mitigates colic and insomnia, and has a calming effect on infants during teething. It enhances the expulsion of gases that may accumulate in the digestive tract, and can be used as an anti-spasmodic.

Saffron has been used thousands of years by therapists and medical practitioners in herbal formulations and ayurvedic (a form of alternative medicine) medicines.

Amongst them: Saffron regulates menstrual disorders. It relieves headaches when applied as a paste to the forehead: it is an anti-depressant, and an aphrodisiac (sexual arousal) for impotency. It also prolongs vitality and is thought to be an anti-aging agent.

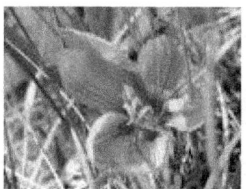 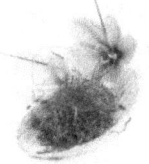

23. <u>Sage</u>: (Salvia officinalis), belongs to the mint family Lamiaceae, having aromatic grayish-green, opposite leaves. Sage is a fragrant herb that can be used for many reasons. Sage has been used throughout history for adding flavor to food, for beauty needs and medicinal purposes.

Sage is a multi-use herb. Sage is an herb that is most often used in cooking and very commonly associated with Thanksgiving holiday stuffing. Sage is a hearty plant that thrives in full sun. Sage can be used as a natural astringent or as an after-shave. Adding sage leaves to your bath and rinse water can enhance dark hair. Sage is also known to help with excess moisture and can be used as an antiperspirant.

Cooking: Sage can be used in savory dishes with pork or sausage and as a flavoring in biscuits and cornbread. Sage's strong smell is often used to mask the aroma of stronger flavored meats such as goose, duck and pork.

Sage is also one of the ingredients used in poultry seasoning. Be advised that sage is strong, and should be used sparingly when cooking, whether using the fresh or dried herb. Plant sage in a pot for cooking or include it in the garden border along with other herbs or near flowers to provide a variety of green, a pleasing fragrance and shape for the flower border. It's resilient and grows well in full sun.

Medicinal properties: Used primarily as a tea, sage can be drunk in moderation to alleviate <u>headaches</u> and <u>sore throats</u> as well as <u>indigestion</u>.

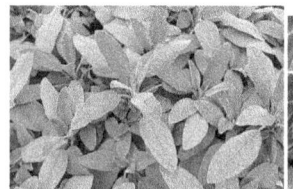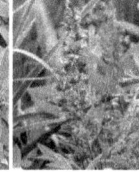

24. **Tarragon**: (Artemisia dracunculus) is a species of perennial herb in the family Asteraceae. One sub-species, Artemisia dracunculus var. sativa, is cultivated for use of the leaves as an aromatic culinary herb. It is considered a shrub related to sunflowers.

The two main types of tarragon are French tarragon and Russian tarragon. The supermarket variety is typically French tarragon, which emits sweet and spicy flavor with hints of fennel and anise. Russian tarragon is the inferior relative to French tarragon. Though its flavor is similar to French tarragon, it's noticeably weaker.

The French use tarragon to flavor everything from chicken Fricassee to Béarnaise sauce. Tarragon is has long, dark green leaves, and it has its best flavor during spring.

Culinary Uses: Tarragon is known for its flavor when combined with white wine vinegar, which preserves its freshness. Some cooks use the leaves and flowers of tarragon as toppings for eggs, fish, shrimp, salad, mushrooms and tomatoes.

Chopped tarragon also adds flavor to condiments such as mustard, mayonnaise, tartar sauce and vinaigrette. Other herbs also benefit from tarragon combinations: the spice enhances the flavors of dill, thyme, garlic and bay leaves.

Medicinal Uses: Tarragon can be used to soothe toothaches as well as used to prevent heart disease. Tarragon for salt can be used to reduce sodium intake for people with hypertension. Tarragon can also be used as a digestive aid to prevent stomach problems and to increase appetite. Tarragon is also a good source of antioxidants.

Tarragon tastes best when consumed fresh. When purchasing tarragon, avoid herbs that appear old or shriveled. Tarragon contains volatile essential oil that's lost when tarragon is dried. Fresh herbs should be stored on the top shelf of the refrigerator: Tarragon lasts up to two weeks refrigerated.

Some cooks keep tarragon in water-filled vases so it stays fresh. Consumers using dried tarragon should make sure the herb doesn't have faded leaves and poor or bad aroma.

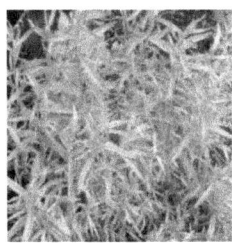 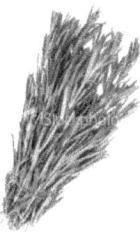 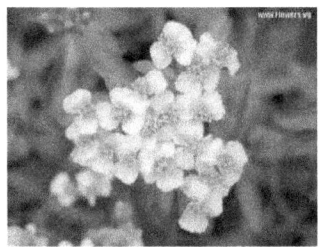

25. Thyme: is any of several species of culinary and medicinal herbs of the genus Thymus, most commonly Thymus vulgaris.

Thyme belongs to the mint family, Lamiaceae. The following is a list of things that thyme is good for whether in the form of an essential oil or a tea taken internally or applied topically.

Thyme:

   relieves aches and muscle and joint pains
   elevates mood and has a calming effect in stress-related
   conditions
   aids in inflammations of the mouth and cures throat
   infections
   useful in the treatment of acute and chronic bronchitis
   aids in treating whooping cough, croup and asthma
   symptoms
   helps to treat inflammation of the upper respiratory tract

possesses terpenoids which are recognized for their <u>cancer preventive</u> properties

relieves chest and respiratory problems including coughs, bronchitis, and chest congestion

expels parasites in the body

useful for easing <u>menstrual cramps</u> and PMS

helps dissolve and remove mucus from the intestinal tract

prevents infection in small wounds

acts as a digestive tonic and <u>increases the appetite</u> and aid in digestion

helps reduce symptoms of irritable bowel and <u>colic</u>

helps in preventing chronic gastritis

excellent against plaque formation and dental decay and gingivitis

relieves <u>sore throat and laryngitis and tonsillitis</u>

heals mouth sores and bad breath (halitosis)

can be used as a poultice for insect bites, <u>stings</u>, mastitis and wounds

cures hookworm, threadworm and roundworm

can also destroy skin parasites like the <u>scabies and lice</u>

effectively fights against bacterial, fungal and <u>viral infections</u>

very effective against Bacillus subtilis, Escherichia coli, and Staphalococcus aureus

helps relax the smooth vessels of the gastrointestinal tract and eases diarrhea

can be used as <u>eyewash</u> to cure sore eyes

can be used as a hair rinse to <u>prevent dandruff</u>

alleviates nervous disorders like nightmares, depression, anxiety, insomnia and melancholy

eases epilepsy and convulsions

protects and increases the quantity of healthy fats found in the cell membranes

can be crushed and used to clean cuts and scrapes, offering an immediate antiseptic remedy

can relieve hangovers

helpful in some cases like Alzheimer's disease, arthritis, athlete's foot, and hair loss

vaginal disease, skin diseases, and reduces scars and other ugly spots on skin

muscle cramps, <u>mosquito repellent</u>
cures conjunctivitis, <u>pink eye</u> and sty.

Warning: Medicinal doses of thyme and especially thyme oil are not recommended during pregnancy as thyme can act as a uterine stimulant.

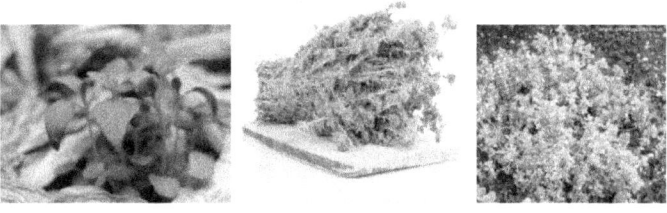

26. <u>Turmeric</u>: (Curcuma longa) is a rhizomatous herbaceous perennial plant of the ginger family, Zingiberaceae. Turmeric, the yellow spice <u>used in curry</u>, is more than just a flavorful addition to a meal. It contains an active nutrients called <u>curcumin</u>, which has been used as a <u>treatment for arthritis and dementia</u>, and which some researchers suspect may be effective in <u>fighting cancer</u>.

Turmeric is a <u>shrub similar to ginger</u>. It is known for both its bitter, <u>mustard like taste</u> and its golden color. Sometimes described as the "<u>poor man's saffron</u>," because of its bright yellow coloring and the fact that it's much more readily available than saffron, turmeric is used in small amounts as a food coloring in dairy products, beverages, cereal, confectionaries, ice cream, bakery items and savory products to obtain a lemon or banana color.

<u>Turmeric is also used to flavor food products such as sausages, pickles, sauces, chutneys, relishes and fish</u>, and it is one of the principal ingredients of curry powder.

 Turmeric can be made into a paste and applied directly to the skin, in paste form, to heal wounds and treat eczema. It can also be used, in paste or powder form, to prevent scarring and scabbing from chicken pox and smallpox.

Turmeric has also been found to be effective in treating arthritis and osteoporosis. That is because turmeric blocks a pathway that affects bone reabsorption. Turmeric may also be effective in treating other inflammatory disorders, including asthma, multiple sclerosis and inflammatory bowel disease.

Turmeric aids the body's ability to digest fat, and it helps relieve gas and bloating. It is also used for other conditions, including heartburn, ulcers and gallstone.

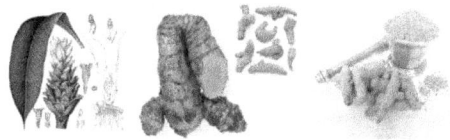

INDEX

FOODS CONTAINING ANTI-OXIDANTS ARE ALSO GOOD ANTI-AGING NUTRIENTS

Vitamin C:
Citrus fruits
Berries
Tomatoes
Peppers
Cabbage
Broccoli
Brussels Sprouts
Cauliflower
Cantaloupe

Vitamin E:
Vegetable oils (wheat germ oil is especially rich in vitamin E)
Wheat and other cereal grains
Green leafy vegetables
Egg yolk
Milk fat
Butter
Meat
Nuts
Organ Meats
Seafood
Avocados

Vitamin A:
Liver
Egg yolks
Whole milk
Carrots
Sweet potato
Kale Turnip greens   Mustard greens
Pink Grapefruit
Broccoli
Cantaloupe

Apricots
Beet greens
Collard greens:
Papaya
Red Peppers
Cheddar cheese

Zinc:
Lean meat
Seafood
Eggs
Green leafy vegetables
Soybeans
Peanuts
Whole Bran
Whole cereals
Cheese
Oysters

Lutein and Zeaxanthin:
Kale
Collard greens
Spinach
Parsley (not dried)
Celery
Broccoli
Lettuce
Green peas
Pumpkin
Brussels sprouts
Summer squash
Corn
Green beans
Green peppers
Cucumbers
Green olives

Note: It is often quoted, "we are what we eat". There is no better way to get healthy and stay healthy than to include anti-inflammatory and anti-oxidant food nutrients in your daily diet.

DETOXIFICATION DIET

(From "The Importance of the Sugar/Fiber Ratio")

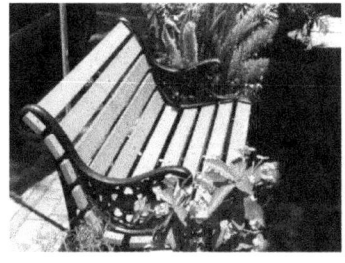

Detoxification has been practiced for centuries by many cultures around the world, including Jews and Christians alike as well as the Chinese medical systems. Detoxification works because it addresses the needs of individual cells. Studies show that everyone would benefit if they detoxed at least once a year. Even a short detoxifying program that just cleanses the liver is beneficial for health.

A full Detoxification diet is about resting, cleaning and nourishing the body from the inside out. Detoxification enhances the body's own natural healing systems. By removing and eliminating toxins from the blood, then feeding your body with healthy nutrients, detoxifying can help protect you from disease, even many cancers and renew your ability to maintain optimum health.

It does this mainly by removing impurities from the blood via the liver, where toxins are detoxified.

The body can then eliminate these "detoxified (neutralized) toxins" through the kidneys, intestines/colon, lungs, lymph and skin. However, when any of these systems are compromised, toxins aren't properly detoxified and every cell in the body is subjected to injury, inflammation and disease.

Toxins are harmful (poisonous) substances and are obstacles to your health and natural healing processes. In order to prevent many of our modern day medical diseases it is necessary to maintain a healthy liver free of sludge.

A detox diet can help your liver's natural cleaning process and eliminating toxins by:

1) Resting your liver, first, through a form of fasting:

2) Stimulating your liver to detoxify:

3) Promoting the elimination of these toxins through the intestines, kidneys and skin:

4) Improving the circulation of the blood:

5) Refueling the body with healthy nutrients.

Remember, your body doesn't detoxify you - it is your liver that detoxifies your body. The liver uses enzymes, vitamins, minerals, anti-oxidants, and anti-inflammatory nutrients to neutralize free radicals. And it is these free radicals that cause most of our medical diseases.

There are many detoxification diets, recipes and programs that depend on your individual needs. There are several programs that stick to a 7-day schedule to ensure the body has enough time to cleanse the blood. When partaking in such a program you might expect to fast on liquids only for two days, with a 5-day 'detox' diet following to give the digestive system time to rest Also, herbs, supplements, low stress exercises, and practices such as dry-skin brushing and hydrotherapy are recommended.

A 3-7 day juice fast is a very strict and effective way to reduce toxins and is considered a very severe form of detoxifying. It involves drinking only fresh fruit and vegetable juices (especially celery and carrot juice) and water.

Other popular detoxifying programs and natural body cleanses include: 1. Cleansing supplement packages, which generally contain fiber, vitamins, herbs and minerals. There are several safe products on the market. 2. A routine of drinking only water one day each week — an ancient practice of many cultures. Drinking only water for one day was a form of fasting in Biblical times.

YOUR LIVER IS RESPONSIBLE FOR DETOXIFING YOUR BODY.

<u>Detoxification is one of the many functions of the liver</u>. Remember: The liver combines toxic substances, such as drugs, alcohol, metabolic waste and environmental toxins with substances such as anti-oxidants, anti-inflammatory nutrients, vitamins and minerals that are not toxic to produce a neutralized substance. This neutralized substance is then excreted through the skin, kidneys and/or intestines (bowel). Certain nutritional drinks and/or foods help cleanse and maintain the liver and then heal many important functions needed by the body to heal and maintain good health.

The best way to get healthy is to work from the inside out starting with the cleansing (detoxification) of the liver. Putting the proper nutrients into your body is always important, but first you want to flush out the toxins.

Toxic chemicals are really poisons. Remember, toxic chemicals cause many of our modern day medical diseases. The toxins that build up in the body are usually noticed first in your skin, causing it to look rough and dull: your body will begin to look puffy and then a disease process begins.

<u>If your system is clean and free</u> of toxic, poisonous chemicals that

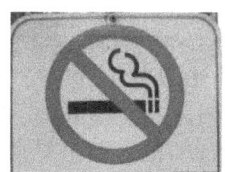

<u>inflame and therefore cause cell damage: then and only then can the good nutrients you put into your body finally get to where they belong</u>. When this finally happens then and only then can you be more energetic, beautiful and healthy. There are many everyday natural foods that are great for detoxifying. **To begin a detox diet you will first need to reduce your toxin load**. To do this you will need to eliminate alcohol, coffee, cigarettes, refined sugars,

especially high fructose corn syrups and artificial sweeteners as well as saturated fats, especially foods that contain trans-fats.

Trans-fats are found in nearly all processed foods on the market today. Trans-fat is another name for hydrogenated oils (margarine, shortening, etc.). And trans-fats are in any food made with these hydrogenated oils. This includes mayonnaise, some ice creams most cookies and/or nearly all processed baked goods. All of the above processed food products contain toxins.

Also, a detox diet works best if you minimize stress. Stress triggers your body to release stress hormones into your system. These hormones, in large amounts, can not only create toxins but also slow down the detoxification enzymes in the liver.

Along with detoxifying your body through diet, it is good to reduce stressful life situations. Yoga, some low stress exercises and meditation are simple and effective ways to relieve stress by resetting your physical and mental reactions to the inevitable stress life will bring.

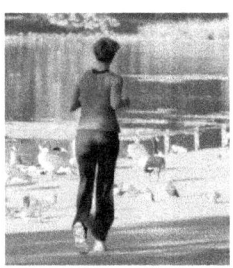

Foods that are known to help the liver detoxify free radicals:

*Celery and/or celery juice. The road to detoxification and therefore the road to healing may start with consuming celery juice. Celery juice is a good one to start with because celery juice has "natural" sodium, i.e. the same content of sodium as human blood (0.09%). If the saline level in your body is not hydrated you can become dehydrated causing hypernatremia: or over-hydrated causing hyponatremia. The salt in celery helps our bodies utilize the nutrients that are put into it.

 The sodium in celery is organic and good for our bodies. Celery deletes carbon dioxide from the body and thereby regulates or counteracts the acid build up in the body. Celery has a great deal of fiber that helps control the absorption of dietary sugars and cholesterol thus controlling the blood sugar and cholesterol levels. Celery also helps the body to regulate temperature.

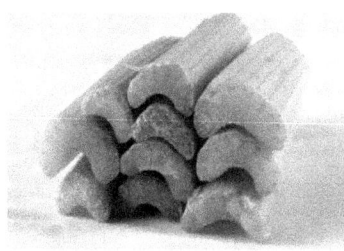

Celery is also good for the colon (digestive system) because it is also a <u>colon cleanser</u>. The nutrients in celery can also stimulate the elimination of urine from the body, and therefore celery acts as a <u>diuretic</u>. Celery is also a calming agent that is good for treating anxiety or other nervous disorders. Celery has been used for its medicinal powers for centuries. It is best to juice celery. However, celery is good cooked in soups and stews or eaten raw in salads. Celery is a food that basically brings the body back to normal.

* Warm Lemon Water: Lemons are a super-food rich in potassium, vitamin C and citric acid. Hot water and lemon, (a lemon tonic), has long been used as a staple in dietary programs for its positive effects on the liver, bile and digestion. Drinking warm lemon water can help cleanse the liver.

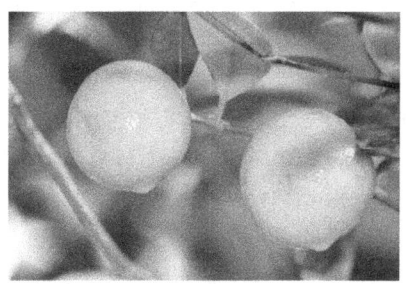

*Dandelion Tea: Dandelion contains nutrients, such as calcium,

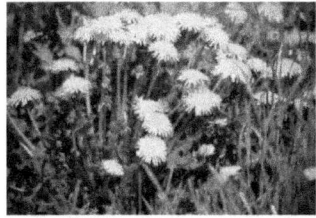

magnesium, iron, selenium, zinc, phosphorous and vitamins B and Dandelions can be boiled into a therapeutic tea that helps cleanses the liver.

*Fruit Smoothies: certain fresh fruits help to stimulate energy flow through the liver, enhancing its function. Blackberries, strawberries, blueberries, raspberries, gooseberries are considered good liver detoxing agents. NOTE- These healthy and potent berries make a delicious liver cleansing fruit smoothie when combined with other fruits, i.e., banana, and/or green leafy vegetables, i.e., spinach and almond milk.

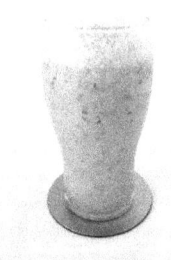

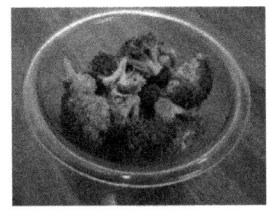

*Broccoli And Cabbage Juice: Broccoli and cabbage are cruciferous vegetables that can be juiced into a cleansing liver drink. Cruciferous vegetables are a rich indoles source. These vegetables include Brussels sprouts, broccoli, bok choy, cabbage and turnips.

Increasing your cruciferous vegetable intake is not recommended if you have a thyroid disorder. Cruciferous vegetables are known as goitrogens, which are foods that can suppress thyroid function. Note- eating a diet rich in fruits, vegetables and cereal grains may help to reduce your risk of cancer as well as other diseases.

*Bananas: Another example of a nutritious medicinal food is the

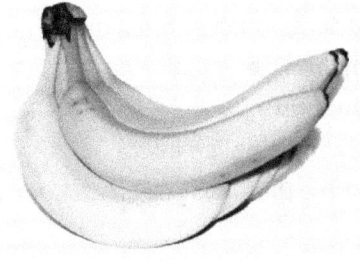

banana. Bananas are one of the most popular foods and for good reason. Bananas are filled with Potassium: giving your body the ability to handle stress, maintain a healthy blood pressure and provide sustained energy - the healthy way without any harmful side effects.

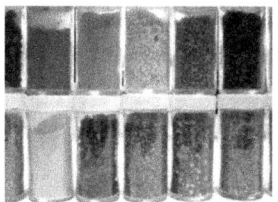

*Nutmeg can also clean your liver and kidney and remove many toxins. Just add nutmeg to as many fruit and milk drinks as you can. You can also add a dash of cinnamon.

A Fruit & Veggie Flush is a 3 day diet that is considered both a detox diet and a weight loss diet that is considered safe for losing 8 to 10 pound. This diet should not be continued after 3 days. During these 3 days, you will only eat fruits and vegetables and drink lots of water: you'll lose weight and conquer food addiction. Basically, this vegetarian diet is really a jump-start diet to a safe and effective weight loss program that includes moderate exercise.

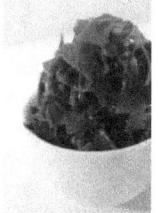

*Seaweed . Seaweed contains a variety of nutrients and minerals, making it an excellent detox food choice. Harmful toxins are removed from the body when they bind with the nutrients.

* Garlic. A well-known blood purifier, garlic is high in detox properties due to the antioxidants it contains. Garlic is also known as a natural cholesterol lowering supplement.

* Apple Cider Vinegar. Long used for its purifying properties, apple cider vinegar is a natural way to purify your body.

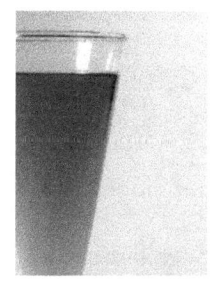

Not only does apple cider vinegar help your body detox, it also supports your immune system, helps control weight and promotes good digestion.

* Spirulina. The spirulina contains many nutrients and can boost nutrition during a detox phase. Dried spirulina contains about 60% (51–71%) protein. It is a complete protein containing all essential amino acids. It is superior to typical plant protein, such as that from legumes.

* High Fiber Raw Fruits and Veggies. Raw fruits and veggies are excellent purifying foods due to the amount of fiber they contain. Fiber is incredibly cleansing when it comes to the digestive system. Many people do not get near enough fiber

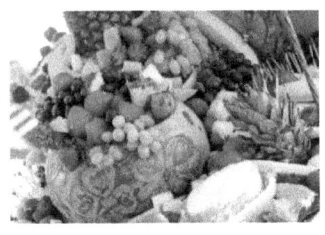

in their daily diet. High fiber fruits and veggies include: apples, arugula, bananas, blackberries, blueberries, carrots, figs, kale and strawberries.

The following are seven key principles to obtain optimal health.

1. Drink 6 to 15 cups (2 to 4 quarts) of pure water daily.

2. Minimize salt intake and maximize your potassium intake.

3. Eat the right types of fats, i.e., omega 3 fatty acids in fish or 1 to 3 grams of fish oil a day

4. Eat limited amounts of meat. Avoid processed meats.

5. Reduce your exposure to pesticides, both internal and external exposure.

6. Eat a wide variety of colorful fruits and vegetables.

7. Get at least 25 to 30 grams of fiber each day.

8. Eat low glycemic carbohydrates (complex carbohydrates) to regulate your blood sugar level.

9. Avoid drinks containing artificial, non-nutritive sweeteners or high fructose corn syrup.

Note- The main strength of a Fruit and Veggie detox diet is that it encourages you to eat fresh fruits and vegetables, which are an essential part of a healthful diet.

BIOGRAPHY   DENISE MARKS, M.D.

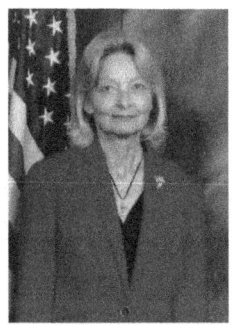

Denise Marks is a retired medical doctor who has renewed her interest in writing and teaching. She specializes in writing about subjects related to medicine, nutrition, health as well as safe and effective means of weight loss. After more than 20 years as a practicing family physician, she has retired to the Mountain Home area of Arkansas to begin a "physician guided weight loss program" that focuses on good nutrition and healthy life style changes that will be beneficial in not only correcting health problems but will also help individuals achieve their ideal weight, a healthier life style and prevent many of today's age-related metabolic medical diseases. For example, it is well documented that being over-weight as well as eating to many empty high caloric simple carbohydrates (i.e., sweet tasting snacks and soda drinks that contain high fructose corn syrup as well as artificial nonnutritive sweeteners) is the number one cause of diabetes, heart disease and/or hypertension which is now known as the "metabolic syndrome". And this syndrome is becoming pandemic in America: mainly due to life styles that involve eating too many sweets (simple carbohydrates) and participating less in physical activity. It has now recognized that eating nutritious foods and maintaining a healthy weight is at the top of the list for preventing or correcting many of these modern day metabolic medical problems.

Born in Billings, Montana, Carla Denise graduated in 1965 from the Huntley Project High School in Worden, Montana. She then joined the U.S. Marine Corps and served from 1965 – 1968. After finishing her military obligation she used the GI Bill to obtain a college education. She received her BS degree in Health and Physical Education with a minor in Chemistry and Biology and began teaching in 1971. She taught school for 7 years in Louisiana. However, when one of her students was accepted into medical school, she realized she could also become a medical doctor. She enjoyed teaching but wanted to help people, one-on-one, with the knowledge she had gained. As a classroom teacher and with class sizes of 24 to 30 students: she felt she was more of a disciplinarian than a teacher.

After obtaining her M.D. degree in 1986 from Louisiana State University Medical Center in Shreveport, LA, she went on in 1988 to receive her

Arkansas medical license. She then moved to Arkansas where she began her medical practice in rural Arkansas, between Dover and Witt Springs. She also worked as an Emergency Room Physician in various small hospitals throughout northern Arkansas from 1995 to 2003. In 1998 she moved her medical practice to the Salem, Horseshoe Bend and Cherokee Village area of Arkansas where she not only kept clinic hours but also continued to work in the Salem and Cherokee Village Hospitals as one of their ER physicians. She also delivered babies at the Salem hospital from 1998 until 2002. This was during the (time) when rural hospitals could obtain malpractice insurance for family physicians doing obstetrics as well as a time that family physicians could afford malpractice in obstetrics.

Her mission still remains "to serve others" by teaching or instructing them on how they can become a healthier individual by using natural (food) nutrients. She believes good nutrition and a healthy weight are at the core of achieving this goal for all individuals. By achieving a healthy weight and eating healthy (food) nutrients, (*avoiding sugar, nonnutritive artificial sweeteners and hydrogenated oils or trans-fats, i.e., margarine and shortening and processed foods made with these "trans-fats"*), she believes individuals can prevent, treat and even cure many of their own health problems.   For example, stress management and poor nutritional eating are known to be risk factors that contribute to arthritis, diabetes, hypertension, heart disease due to high cholesterol/high triglyceride eye disease, anxiety, depression, acid reflux (GERD), neurological diseases and chronic pain issues, etc. Knowledge, about good nutrition and safe and effective weight loss as well as how to handle stress, will be the center of focus at each encounter.

Dr. Marks is the proud and happy mother of 2 adult sons as well as a grandmother. She is also a proud Marine veteran and an active a member of Twin Lakes Marines and the Marine Corps League. As a veteran of the Vietnam era she continues to help veterans, through diet, counseling and medication, who deal with post traumatic issues and depression, overcome some of the issues that hinder them from achieving a better quality of life.

DENISE MARKS, M.D.

www.ingramcontent.com/pod-product-compliance
Lightning Source LLC
Chambersburg PA
CBHW070643290526
45790CB00001B/180